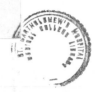
19

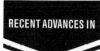

Ophthalmology

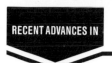

Ophthalmology

Edited by

S. I. Davidson FRCS FCOphth DO
Formerly Director of Studies, Department of
Ophthalmology, University of Liverpool;
Surgeon, St Paul's Eye Hospital,
Liverpool; Consultant Neuro-ophthalmologist,
Walton Hospital, Liverpool, UK

B. Jay MD FRCS FCOphth
Professor of Clinical Ophthalmology,
Institute of Ophthalmology, University
of London, London, UK

NUMBER EIGHT

CHURCHILL LIVINGSTONE
EDINBURGH LONDON MELBOURNE NEW YORK AND TOKYO 1992

CHURCHILL LIVINGSTONE
Medical Division of Longman Group UK Limited

Distributed in the United States of America by Churchill
Livingstone Inc., 650 Avenue of the Americas, New York,
N.Y. 10011, and by associated companies, branches and
representatives throughout the world.

First published 1992

ISBN 0-443-04373-6
ISSN 0309 2437

British Library Cataloguing in Publication Data
A catalogue record for this book is
available from the British Library

Library of Congress Cataloging in Publication Data is
available

Produced by Longman Singapore Publishers Pte Ltd
Printed in Singapore

Preface

The increasing subspecialization in ophthalmology has made it difficult for the practising ophthalmologist to be conversant with advances in the specialty that continue to occur at an accelerating rate. Indeed, coping with the current literature of one's specialist interest is arduous. Accordingly, in order to keep this volume to manageable proportions our choice of subject has necessarily been selective.

Some of the remarkable advances that have been made in ophthalmology over the past decade are mirrored in the breadth of topics covered in this issue. The basic sciences are represented by chapters on Uveitis by Forrester and Molecular genetics in clinical ophthalmology by Jay and Jay. Surgical advances in the past two decades are illustrated by Oculoplastic surgery by Beaconsfield and Collins, Corneal graft failure by Pendergrast and colleagues, Complications of intraocular lenses by Steele, Cryotherapy of retinopathy of prematurity by Fielder and Pneumatic retinopexy by Brinton and Hilton. Medical ophthalmology is represented by the chapter on Contact lens practice by Buckley and Morris, Medical versus surgical treatment of primary open angle glaucoma by Jay and charged particle irradiation of melanoma of the choroid by Char and Castro. The application of modern technology to methods of investigation is amply demonstrated in the chapter on Automated perimetry by Wishart.

We hope that by presenting such diverse topics, the interest of ophthalmologists at all stages in their careers will be attracted, from those at the beginning of their training to ophthalmic surgeons of many years' standing.

Liverpool   S.I.D.
London   B.J.
1992

Contributors

W. J. Armitage BSc PhD
Senior Research Fellow, Department of Ophthalmology, University of
Bristol, Bristol, UK

M. Beaconsfield FRCS FCOphth DO
Senior Registrar, Moorfields Eye Hospital, London, UK

Daniel A. Brinton MD
Assistant Clinical Professor, Department of Ophthalmology, University of
California, San Francisco, USA

R. Buckley FRCS FCOphth
Director, Contact Lens and Prosthesis Department, Moorfields Eye
Hospital, London, UK

Joseph R. Castro MD
Professor and Vice Chairman, Radiation Oncology, University of
California, San Francisco, USA

Devron H. Char MD
Professor, Departments of Ophthalmology, Radiation Oncology and the
Francis I. Proctor Foundation, and Director, Ocular Oncology Unit,
University of California; Consultant, San Francisco General Hospital, and
Fort Miley VA Hospital, San Francisco, USA

J. R. O. Collin FRCS
Consultant Surgeon, Moorfields Eye Hospital; Honorary Consultant
Ophthalmic Surgeon, Hospital for Sick Children, Great Ormond Street,
London, UK

David L. Easty MD FRCS FCOphth
Professor of Ophthalmology, and Head, Department of Ophthalmology,
University of Bristol, UK

A. R. Fielder FRCS FCOphth
Professor of Ophthalmology, University of Birmingham Medical School,
Birmingham, UK

J. V. Forrester MD FRCS(E) FRCS(G)
Cockborn Professor of Ophthalmology, University of Aberdeen, Aberdeen, UK

George F. Hilton MD
Clinical Professor and Co-Director of the Retina Service, Department of Ophthalmology, University of California, San Francisco, USA

Barrie Jay MD FRCS FCOphth
Professor of Clinical Ophthalmology, Institute of Ophthalmology, University of London, London, UK

Marcelle Jay PhD
Senior Lecturer in Ophthalmic Genetics, Institute of Ophthalmology, University of London, London, UK

Jeffrey L. Jay BSc MB ChB FRCS FCOphth
Honorary Senior Lecturer, University of Glasgow; Consultant Ophthalmologist, Western Infirmary, Glasgow, UK

Judith Morris FBCO
Optometrist, Contact Lens and Prosthesis Department, Moorfields Eye Hospital, London, UK

D. G. C. Pendergrast FRACO FRACS
Clinical Research Fellow, Department of Ophthalmology, University of Bristol, Bristol, UK

Chris A. Rogers BSc PhD
Biostatistician and Data Manager, United Kingdom Transplant Service, Bristol, UK

Arthur D. McG. Steele FRCS FRACO FCOphth DO
Consultant Surgeon, Moorfields Eye Hospital, London, UK

Andy Vail BSc MSc
Biostatistician, United Kingdom Transplant Service, Bristol, UK

P. K. Wishart MBChB FRCS(G) FCOphth DO
Consultant Ophthalmic Surgeon, St Paul's Eye Hospital, Liverpool, UK

Contents

1

Oculoplastic surgery

M. Beaconsfield   J. R. O. Collin

INTRODUCTION

Plastic and reconstructive lid surgery is hailed as a new and growing subspecialty in ophthalmology. Some concepts, however, have roots in antiquity: everting sutures for entropion were used in the time of Hippocrates.

Recent advances in oculoplastic surgery are in the main technical and not all aspects can be covered in one chapter. Most of these fall into three categories and representative examples of each are discussed: adaptations of well-tried procedures from other surgical specialties (Mersilene and osseointegration), the rediscovery of an old treatment (cryosurgery) and the 'new' use of an old established technique (micrographic surgery).

MERSILENE

Synthetic meshes have been used successfully for several years to correct defects such as diaphragmatic or abdominal hernias (Adler & Furne 1959, Bailey & Love 1988), as slings in urological and gynaecological repair (Nichols 1973), in tendon reconstruction (Amis 1982), for sternotomy closure in cardiothoracic operations (Johnston et al 1985, Sirivella et al 1987) and in spinal surgery (Gaines & Abernathie 1986). Their mechanical properties and porosity have been documented (Chu & Wech 1985).

Mersilene in particular is proving to be useful in oculoplastic surgery as a sling for brow suspensions (Downes & Collin 1989) instead of fascia lata, and as a spacer for lid retraction in dysthyroid eye disease instead of sclera (Downes & Jordan 1989).

Mersilene is available as a mesh and consists of interlocking polyester fibres. It is manufactured by a knitting-machine process which interlocks each individual fibre, thus preventing unravelling (Ethicon 1985, Mersilene mesh product sheet). It can therefore be cut to whatever size or shape is necessary. Like cloth, Mersilene has a bias, i.e. it gives when pulled in one direction but not at 90° to it (Fig. 1.1). Thus, if being cut for strips, it is important to do so along its non-stretching axis. Equally, if used as a spacer for dysthyroid lid retraction, the Mersilene graft must be placed in the lid with the non-stretching axis in the vertical direction.

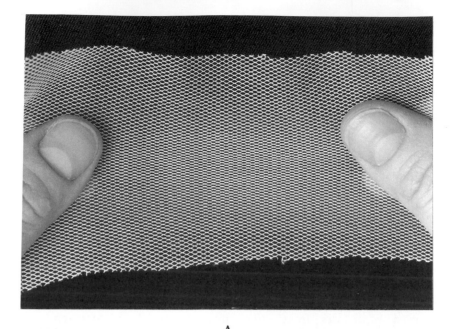

Fig. 1.1 **A** Mersilene sheet resisting stretch in one direction. **B** Mersilene sheet 'giving' at 90° to **A**.

Brow suspension

Ptosis surgery, depending on the degree of lid drop and the amount of levator function, has been well established into three techniques: the Fasanella–Servat procedure of Muller–tarsoconjunctival resection in mild cases; levator resection (anterior or posterior approach) in moderate cases and brow suspension in severe cases (Waller et al 1987).

The congenital absence or near absence of a skin crease in the upper lid is the first evidence of poor levator function and under these circumstances one must resort to the frontalis muscle as the elevator. A number of different materials have been used as slings in the past, such as various surgical sutures (Friedenwald & Guyton 1948, Katowitz 1979), silicone (Tillett & Tillett 1966), sclera (Bodian 1968), and even orbicularis muscle strips on pedicles, all with disappointing results. Fascia lata (autogenous or stored) has been used for several years with much better and longer-lasting results (Crawford 1977). The harvesting of fascia from the patient's leg has its own complications and may not be possible (e.g. the child is too young and therefore his leg is not long enough) or desirable (e.g. general anaesthesia inappropriate). Furthermore, stored fascia may not be readily available. Mersilene offers a suitable alternative.

A brow suspension using Mersilene is done under general anaesthetic in children and local anaesthetic in adults. Mersilene strips are cut approximately 5–7 mm wide and 15 cm long. These are autoclaved and packaged prior to use. When required, they are soaked on the instrument trolley in a suitable antibiotic solution for about 10 minutes and then thoroughly rinsed in sterile saline prior to insertion.

Five horizontal stab incisions are made in a modified Fox pentagon (Collin 1989). A lid guard is placed under the lid to protect the globe (Fig. 1.2). The two horizontal eyelid stab incisions are made through skin and orbicularis 3–7 mm from the eyelid margin to match the position of the lid crease in the fellow lid. If doing a bilateral procedure, the surgeon chooses the level most cosmetically acceptable. These lid incisions are placed at the junctions of the medial and central third, and the central and lateral third of the lid. The medial and lateral brow incisions are made just within the superior hairline of the brow, slightly in from the level of the medial and lateral canthus, respectively. The superior brow incision is made halfway between these two at about 10 mm above the brow. The three brow incisions are made deep to the level of periosteum and the profuse bleeding that naturally ensues is controlled by pressure.

The strips are threaded through in the same manner as for fascia lata, with a Wright's fascial needle, taking care to remain superficial to the tarsal plate but deep to orbicularis (Fig. 1.3). The two ends of the mesh are brought out of the superior brow incision, pulled tight until the required lid height is achieved and secured with a 5.0 ethibond suture through the mesh just inside

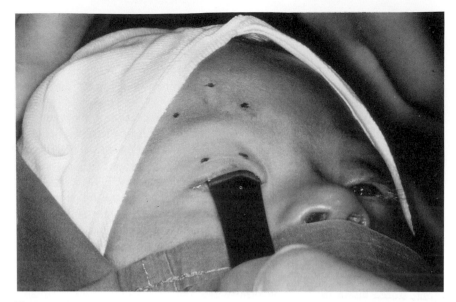

Fig. 1.2   Metal lid guard in situ to protect globe and prospective needle entry points inked on skin.

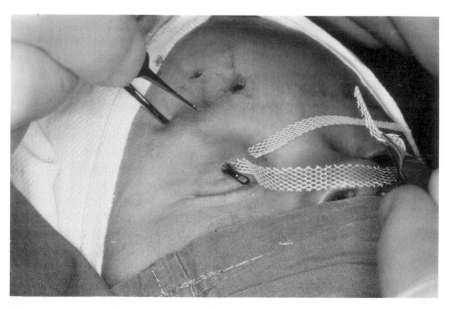

Fig. 1.3   Insertion of Mersilene strip with Wright's fascial needle.

the brow incision. Tying the mesh into a knot makes it too bulky and increases its chances of extrusion.

The excess sling is trimmed and the now secured ends allowed to drop down into the superior brow incision. The three brow incisions are closed with a 6.0 vicryl or nylon suture depending on whether the patient will tolerate suture removal (Fig. 1.4). It is not necessary to suture the lid stab wounds. Topical and systemic antibiotics are routinely prescribed for ten days postoperatively and eye lubrication in the form of drops by day and ointment by night should be continued for a minimum of six months.

Downes & Collin (1989) have described successful results in 17 ptotic lids corrected with Mersilene slings. All maintained their new lid height. Only one postoperative infection occurred, which was successfully treated with systemic antibiotics and did not require removal of the sling. Interestingly, the patient had an unsuspected intercurrent upper respiratory infection at the time of surgery and the patient was inadvertently allowed home without his routine course of oral and topical antibiotics. The average follow-up was ten weeks and a recent review of these patients in clinic has found them to have remained stable and satisfactory.

Lid spacer

Lagophthalmos, corneal exposure and a cosmetically unacceptable wide-eyed look result from lid retraction in dysthyroid eye disease. Several approaches to retractor lengthening have been devised. Henderson (1965) recommended making an incision at the retrotarsal margin through Muller's muscle and portions of the levator aponeurosis, depending on the degree of lid retraction. Bank sclera has been popular for lengthening retractors (Flannagan 1974) but its unpredictable absorption can lead to repeat operations (Dryden & Soll 1977).

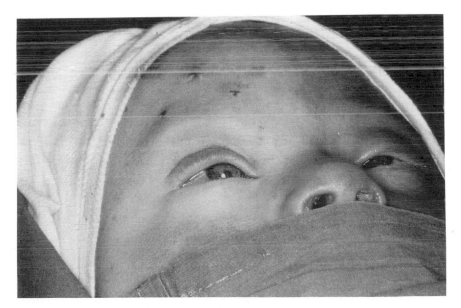

Fig. 1.4 Final per operative appearance with forehead wounds closed with 6.0 vicryl.

Mersilene has recently been shown to produce good cosmetic results as a graft instead of sclera in the treatment of scleral show of dysthyroid origin. The Mersilene is positioned and sutured in a similar way to sclera to lengthen the posterior lamella vertically. In contrast to sclera, less Mersilene seems to be required for the same effect; the postoperative inflammatory response is less aggressive and usually does not require any treatment.

The recommendations for the precise measurements of Mersilene mesh as a lid spacer are described by Downes & Jordan (1989), and are shown in Tables 1.1 and 1.2. Their results show that in four upper and ten lower dysthyroid lids a significant improvement in lid position was achieved. The new eyelid height has been maintained in all patients, whose average follow-up was nine months. Perhaps more importantly, every patient without exception remains delighted with their cosmetic result.

Table 1.1 Upper lid Mersilene dimensions

1.5 × scleral show medially and centrally
2 × scleral show laterally
Horizontal length = tarsus
Eye pads + upper lid traction suture, 48 hours
Topical + oral antibiotics

Table 1.2 Lower lid Mersilene dimensions

1.5 × scleral show
Horizontal length = tarsus
Medial and lateral Frost sutures, 72 hours
Eye pads, 48 hours
Full-thickness bolster sutures, 10–14 days
Topical + oral antibiotics

Inert non-absorbable meshes theoretically provide a scaffold for granulation tissue to grow into and surround. Carbon-fibre materials fragment from about three months (Amis 1982). Gortex is hydrophobic and has a negative surface charge, which may inhibit the incorporation of fibrovascular material. This would not only explain its widespread use in vascular surgery but also its easy extrusion, contrary to Mersilene, when the tissues covering it break down (Karesh et al 1989). It is also comparatively expensive.

Nylon loses its strength after implantation, produces less regular collagen adhesions than polyester, and breaks. This tendency to break has been experienced by many who use it for wound closure in cataract surgery (Richards et al 1988) and some now advocate the use of Mersilene sutures as an alternative.

Mersilene is relatively cheap, readily available, easy to use and incorporates well into the tissues. This of course may be a disadvantage when trying to remove it in the event of extrusion or infection. To date, these complications have been rare. The incorporation of Mersilene into the host tissue has been documented in both animal and clinical studies (Adler & Furne 1959, Amis

1982, Lisman & Smith 1987). Its use in a Fox pentagon allows subsequent insertion of fascia using the Crawford method should this be necessary, as the incisions are different (Collin 1989).

The disadvantages of Mersilene are that it is a foreign material requiring postoperative antibiotic cover, and that further long-term studies will need to confirm the initial favourable results. These are presently being undertaken.

CRYOSURGERY

Injury due to cold has been recognized from the earliest times (Shephard & Dawber 1982). Alexander the Great's troops are believed to have used sesame juice rubbed into their skin for protection against severe cold and, more recently, Napoleon's disastrous Russian campaign gave rise to medical observations on frostbite.

The deliberate destruction of diseased tissue by cold in a controlled manner dates from the nineteenth century when suitable refrigerants became available, such as salt/ice mixtures (Arnott 1851), carbon dioxide snow, liquid air (White 1899, Whitehouse 1907, Puscy 1907) and liquid nitrogen.

After the reintroduction of liquid nitrogen by Zacarian, this refrigerant was adopted by dermatologists in the management of basal and squamous cell carcinoma (Zacarian 1969, 1972, Torre 1971, Lubritz 1977) as well as benign lesions.

Cryosurgery has gained slow acceptance in ophthalmology in the treatment of skin tumours. Recently it has gained popularity because the cure rates and cosmetic results are comparable to other modes of therapy (Beard 1975, Fraunfelder et al 1977), and its use does not necessitate an inpatient stay. It has been reported as a valuable alternative to surgery or radiotherapy, with cure rates approaching 95% (Zacarian 1977, Biro et al 1982, Albright 1982, McIntosh et al 1983, Ashby et al 1989). Among a series of 395 selected non-melanoma skin cancers treated with cryosurgery and followed up for five years, Holt (1988) reports a cure rate of 97%. Recurrences were seen in 6 out of 225 treated basal cell carcinomas at a median time of 18 months; 1 out of 34 squamous cell carcinomas recurred at six months postoperatively and 1 out of 128 Bowen's tumour, also at six months. Other reports are less favourable (Hall et al 1986).

Carcinoma of the skin is the most common malignancy in man. Early detection with effective treatment gives a high cure rate. Its association with areas exposed to sunlight is well documented, as is its recurrence in these cases (Victorian Cancer Registry 1983, Giles et al 1988). Eyelid carcinomas are the same histologically as other facial varieties. However, they do have a predilection for the lid margin, where surgical excision necessitates plastic repair and irradiation can cause cicatricial complications. These lesions are potentially destructive and, if unchecked, can invade and kill. Indeed Birge (1938) reported more than a 10% mortality rate in advanced cases and suggested that upper lid and inner canthal tumours were the worst. This has been confirmed in later works (Aurora & Blodi 1970). A recent review from the Mayo Clinic (Bartley et al 1989) showed that over the last 20 years more than half of the patients presenting for orbital exenteration had extensions due to either basal or squamous cell carcinoma (Bartley et al 1989).

With the increasing emphasis on cost and efficiency, cryosurgery is beginning to gain favour amongst ophthalmologists with an oculoplastic interest. However, it is not a panacea and its misuse might lead to disrepute and its being abandoned as a useful and appropriate mode of treatment in the management of certain lid skin carcinomas.

Those who regularly use this form of treatment recommend that certain rules of case selection for cryosurgery should be adhered to. Other treatment modalities must be examined if:

1.   The tumour is larger than 10 mm or sclerotic in nature
2.   Its margins are not clinically definable
3.   It is fixed to periosteum
4.   It involves conjunctiva
5.   The tumour is pigmented
6.   The patient is pigmented.

Cryosurgery is particularly useful in patients with multiple small basal cell carcinomas where total surgical excision is not technically feasible in terms of plastic repair of the defects, and also where patients with small squamous cell carcinomas are not sufficiently fit for general anaesthesia.

Treatment methods vary in detail, but in principle liquid nitrogen is delivered using a hand-held open spray technique. A cone spray technique and high-performance nitrogen cryo unit with a closed probe are also available (Torre 1977, Faber et al 1990).

After local anaesthetic infiltration, the tumour is outlined with a 5 mm margin and the skin beyond is protected with tape such as blenderm or micropore. When treating the lid, the eye is protected with a temperature-resistant guard such as a plastic coffee spoon, after instillation of topical anaesthetic drops. Thermocouple needles are introduced under the area to be treated; the liquid nitrogen spray tip is held at about 1 cm from the centre of the lesion and spraying is maintained until the desired temperature is reached ($-30°C$ to $-35°C$). A double freeze/thaw cycle is usually employed with time given between the two freezes for complete defrosting of the treated area.

Patients are warned in advance that post-treatment pain can be quite severe for several hours and should be managed with regular analgesia. Oedema and serous discharge from the skin take several days to subside, with sloughing of the epidermis several weeks later. Haemorrhage is unusual.

After treatment to lid lesions the eye is lubricated and firmly padded for 24 hours. This is in an effort to minimize swelling, which can be quite severe as lid skin is lax compared to the rest of the face. Lesions treated beyond the lids (e.g. temple, forehead, cheek) are left uncovered.

The side effects and complications reflect cellular injury due to freezing. Pigment cells are affected first (– 10°C), followed by hair follicles (– 20°C) and basal cells (– 30°C). According to Mazur (1970) the extent of tissue damage depends on the speed at which freezing takes place, how long freezing is maintained, the lowest temperature reached and the rate of thawing. It is now believed that the thawing part of the cycle causes more damage than the freezing. Repeating the cycle causes greater destruction.

A hypertrophic reaction is common and usually resolves within six to eight weeks. Alopecia and depigmentation are usual and patients are informed of this beforehand. If on review there is no lash loss or depigmentation the treatment has not been effective. Depigmentation can be particularly unsightly and although repigmentation occurs to a certain extent over several months, it is never sufficient to match adjacent skin. For this reason cryosurgery is avoided in pigmented patients as the cosmetic result can look worse than the original lesion.

Shephard (1979) has demonstrated that the collagen scaffold of the dermis remains relatively undamaged by freezing at temperatures reached in clinical practice. This explains the rare occurrence of cicatricial deformities. Lid notching is a sign of overtreatment as it indicates necrosis of the tarsal plate.

The lacrimal drainage system also seems to be relatively impervious to freezing at clinical temperatures and cryosurgery should therefore be seriously considered as a treatment option where lacrimal patency is to be saved in the presence of a medial canthal tumour (Caujolle et al 1989).

Trial and error, with accurate observation of side effects and complications, has resulted in – 30 to – 35°C being the recommended temperature range to be achieved for the destruction of common cutaneous cancers. When dealing with malignancies we advocate the use of thermocouple needles to monitor temperature rather than an arbitrary 30-second double freeze/thaw cycle without temperature monitoring as proposed by Holt (1988).

Correct selection of patients with skin cancer for treatment by this method is important and will depend on the experience of the operator. Cryosurgical technique is easy to learn from someone who uses this method routinely but sophisticated enough that unsupervised juniors can have unacceptable complications (Fraunfelder et al 1980). Because it is new to ophthalmology it will probably remain a controversial modality for the foreseeable future.

Nevertheless, the safety, speed, effectiveness and low cost together with excellent clinical and cosmetic results should not continue to be ignored.

MICROGRAPHIC SURGERY

Despite the well-established records of radiotherapy and cryosurgery, many ophthalmologists, given a free choice, would still opt for surgery as the initial treatment for the management of skin carcinomas. It should be the treatment of choice for certain tumours particularly if the patient is young and healthy or if the tumour has recurred at the primary site. Although cure rates are comparable (Gladstein 1978, Fraunfelder et al 1980, Rodriguez–Sains & Jakobiec 1987), many still advocate an aggressive initial approach for total tumour eradication.

Preoperative histological confirmation of clear edges is essential to keep surgical excision to a minimum and, until recently, frozen section control has been the only available method in the UK. With this conventional method, only a small area of the periphery is actually examined microscopically. Standard frozen section examination is incomplete compared to Mohs' micrographic technique and can consume valuable theatre time.

The microscopic examination of fresh tissue as whole layers until all the edges and base are clear was first devised by Frederic Mohs 50 years ago (Mohs 1941). The original technique was preceded and followed by chemical treatment of the tumour and its base and the defect was allowed to heal by second intention. This resulted in some unsightly scarring with disturbance of function, though the cure rate has been shown to have remained high even on long-term follow-up (Mohs 1976).

Mohs' 30-year series of 2563 basal cell carcinomas only had 12 recurrences, 7 of which were successfully treated by repetition of the same method; of 615 squamous cell carcinomas there were 5 recurrences of which 4 were successfully retreated. Tromovitch & Stegeman (1974) reported 3 recurrences in 102 basal cell carcinomas with a follow-up of three to eight years.

It was the unsatisfactory cosmetic results, together with the fact that most of Mohs' trainees were dermatologists, which prevented this technique becoming popular amongst reconstructive and, more specifically, oculoplastic surgeons. Furthermore, specialists trained in the microscopically controlled excision and examination of tumours are not widely available.

This method has now been adopted by the senior author, followed by formal surgical reconstruction rather than laissez-faire, and the preliminary results confirm its value (Anderson & Ceilley 1978, Downs et al 1990).

Technique

The surgical area is prepared in the usual way and the tumour limits are marked with a sterile pen. The area is infiltrated with local anaesthetic and the obvious tumour mass excised in its entirety, including a small margin of normal tissue. Then, a thin layer of tissue, approximately 2 mm thick, is excised from the entire base and edges of the defect. Pressure is applied to produce haemostasis.

This 2-mm thick specimen is divided into quadrants or into convenient portions on a glass slide. The edges of the specimens are colour-coded with red and blue dyes to aid in the precise localization of any remaining carcinoma. Frozen sections are obtained from the undersurface of each specimen. A map is drawn and the exact location of residual carcinoma carefully marked on the map. The process is repeated only in those locations and is continued until the entire area is free. The base is cleaned with hydrogen peroxide and then dressed with tulle gras and a pressure pad.

This micrographic technique employs accurate segmental tissue mapping to avoid the excision of normal tissue. This is particularly important where tumours are large, recurrent, in the medial canthal area where the lacrimal drainage system might be spared, and the eyelid skin where the posterior lamella may be preserved, thus facilitating reconstruction. In all these circumstances, the accurate sparing of normal tissues makes reconstruction easier, while affording the best possible long-term cure.

The disadvantages include the need for a specialist well versed in the technique; the patient may not wish to have or may not tolerate this procedure under local anaesthetic; adequate anaesthesia is often difficult in areas scarred by previous treatment; it is time consuming and with large tumours the examination may take several hours to complete. This is tiring for the surgeon as well as for the patient.

Most tumour studies publish a five-year follow-up; yet tumours can recur after a tumour-free period in excess of that time. On the other hand there have been reports of cure, despite some cases having histologically proved incomplete excisions (Aurora & Blodi 1970, Gooding et al 1965). However, it has been recognized that non-surgical modalities which cannot guarantee tumour-free margins are also effective and it is suggested that an enhanced immunological response as a result of treatment is in part responsible for suppression of the tumour extensions that survive the treatment (Soanes et al 1969, Neel et al 1973).

In the final analysis it may be that five years is insufficient time for accurate comparison of follow-up studies.

Mohs' technique is presently the most efficacious manner to eradicate tumour and has excellent very long-term follow-up results (Mohs 1978). However, it may not be the most efficient when looking at parameters other than long-term cure rate. Nevertheless it offers maximal assurance of eradication with minimum loss of normal tissue. It is therefore suggested as appropriate for large tumours, where reconstruction may be difficult if not enough normal tissue is spared, in recurrent tumours, in the medial canthal area and in lid skin.

The two-step procedure of micrographic excision, followed by repair a day or so later, gives the surgeon time to plan the best possible reconstruction, knowing with confidence that the defect is clear of tumour and that his operating time under general anaesthetic will be kept to the minimum possible.

OSSEOINTEGRATION

Post-exenteration cosmetic rehabilitation is difficult, though spectacle-mounted prostheses can be highly acceptable (Fig. 1.5). Increasingly patients, particularly in the younger age-group, are keen to have orbital prostheses

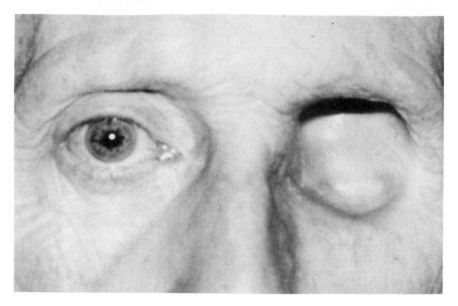

A

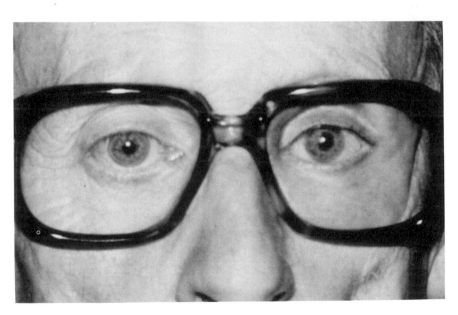

B

Fig. 1.5 **A** Orbital exenteration in a 72-year-old man. **B** Same patient with spectacle-borne prosthesis.

which can be fixed with adhesive, thus obviating glasses. The disadvantage is that adhesive is an irritant to the skin. Furthermore, skin which has received radiotherapy can be intolerant to it.

Tissue-integrated prostheses have been successfully used for several years in clinical dentistry to help edentulous patients who cannot tolerate dentures. Recently, this technique has been adapted to rehabilitate patients who have suffered trauma with organ loss such as an ear, or cancer surgery (Albrektsson et al 1987).

To date titanium is the material most adept at integrating into bone without exciting a fibrous response, and as a result has become the material of choice for bone-fixed implants.

The surgery for the placement of the titanium pegs is done in two stages. First, the titanium pegs are screwed into the bone, after which the overlying periosteum and skin are allowed to heal; several months later the superficial part of the pegs is then exposed to the skin surface and their cover removed to be replaced by the abutments, responsible for fixating the prosthesis. These remain exposed, though covered by small caps during the healing process.

A prosthesis is manufactured to the specifications of each patient, to ensure the best possible skin and eye colour match. The prosthesis can be fixed in a variety of ways to facilitate easy placement and removal of the prosthesis from the orbital pegs by the patient (Fig. 1.6).

The procedure is time consuming and not without risk, and the necessary equipment is expensive. The technique is presently still in its infancy as far as post-exenteration cases are concerned, which is why results cannot be presented at this stage; but refinement and alterations to the original technique are already being done and we hope the coming years will produce encouraging results.

CONCLUSION

Appearance is important and patients now require and demand to live a relatively normal life after major surgery. With the advent of improved and new materials like Mersilene to correct lid ptosis or lid retraction, a better eyelid contour and height can be achieved, resulting in an improved facial appearance. Cryosurgery aims to produce a better cosmetic result by destroying the tumour without removing any tissue at all. Mohs' technique plans to remove the minimum tissue commensurate with complete eradication of the tumour, and osseointegration achieves as normal a life and countenance as possible for patients after major mutilating surgery.

Public awareness and patient pressure will ensure we constantly review our clinical habits, hone old techniques to suit the present and develop new ones to produce as functional and cosmetically acceptable a result as possible.

As Aristotle said (Addison 1711), a good face is a better recommendation than any letter of introduction.

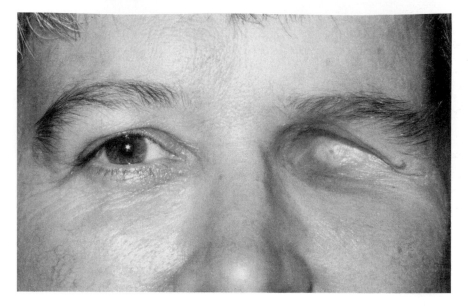

A

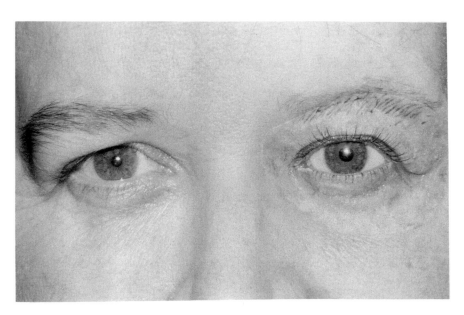

B

Fig. 1.6 A Orbital exenteration with good lid skin preservation in a 44-year-old woman. **B** Same patient with osseointegrated prosthesis. (Reproduced by kind permission of Mr R. Downes.)

REFERENCES

Addison J 1711 The Spectator: 13 November

Adler R H, Furne C N 1959 Use of pliable synthetic mesh in the repair of hernias and tissue defects. Surg Gynecol Obstet 108: 199–206

Albrektsson T, Branemark P I, Jacobsson M et al 1987 Present clinical applications of osseointegrated percutaneous implants. Plast Reconstr Surg 79: 721–730

Albright S D 1982 Treatment of skin cancer using multiple modalities. J Am Acad Dermatol 7: 143–171

Amis A A 1982 Filamentous implant reconstruction of tendon defects: a comparison between carbon and polyester fibres. J Bone Joint Surg [Br] 643–682

Anderson R L, Ceilley R I 1978 A multi-specialty approach to the excision and reconstruction of eyelid tumours. Ophthalmology 85: 1150–1163

Arnott J 1851 On the treatment of cancer by the regulated application of an anaesthetic temperature. Churchill, London

Ashby M A, Smith J, Ainslie J et al 1989 Treatment of non-melanotic skin cancer at a large Australian centre. Cancer 63: 1863–1871

Aurora A L, Blodi F C 1970 Reappraisal of basal cell carcinoma of the eyelids. Am J Ophthalmol 70: 329–336

Bailey H H, Love R J M 1988 Short practice of surgery. Lewis, London pp 1172–1173

Bartley G B, Garrity J A, Waller R R et al 1989 Orbital exenteration at the Mayo Clinic. Ophthalmology 96: 468–474

Beard C 1975 Observations on the treatment of basal cell carcinoma of the eyelids. Trans Am Acad Ophthalmol Otolaryngol 79: 664–670

Birge H L 1938 Cancer of the eyelids: basal cell carcinoma and mixed basal cell and squamous cell epithelioma. Arch Ophthalmol 19: 700–708

Biro L, Price E, Brand A 1982 Cryosurgery for basal cell carcinoma of the eyelids and nose: a 5 year experience. J Am Acad Dermatol 6: 1042–1047

Bodian M 1968 Repair of ptosis using human sclera. Am J Ophthalmol 65: 352–358

Caujolle J P, Clevy J P, Ortonne J P et al 1989 Cryosurgery in the management of eyelid basal cell carcinomas. J Fr Ophthalmol 12: 279–286

Chu C C, Wech L 1985 Characterisation of morphologic and mechanical properties of surgical mesh fabrics. J Biomed Mater Res 19: 903–916

Collin J R O 1989 A manual of systematic eyelid surgery. Churchill Livingstone, Edinburgh

Crawford J S 1977 Repair of ptosis using frontalis muscle and fascia lata: a 20 year review. Ophthalmic Surg 8: 31–40

Downes R N, Collin J R O 1989 The Mersilene mesh sling: a new concept in ptosis surgery. Br J Ophthalmol 73: 498–501

Downes R N, Jordan K 1989 The surgical management of dysthyroid related retraction using Mersilene mesh. Eye 3: 385–390

Downes R N, Walker N P J, Collin J R O 1990 Micrographic (Mohs') surgery in the management of periocular basal cell epitheliomas. Eye 4: 160–168

Dryden R M, Soll D B 1977 The use of scleral transplantation in cicatricial entropion and eyelid retraction. Trans Am Acad Ophthalmol Otolaryngol 83: 669–674

Faber W R, Flinterman J, Mekkes J R 1990 Cryosurgical treatment of basal cell carcinoma of the eyelid. Ned Tijdschr Geneeskd 134: 1002–1005

Flanagan J C 1974 Eye bank sclera in oculoplastic surgery. Ophthalmic Surg 5: 45–53

Fraunfelder F T, Wallis T R, Farris H E et al 1977 The role of cryosurgery in external ocular and periocular disease. Trans Am Acad Ophthalmol Otolaryngol 83: 713–724

Fraunfelder F T, Zacarian S A, Limmer B L et al 1980 Cryosurgery for malignancies of the eyelid. Ophthalmology 87: 461–465

Friedenwald J S, Guyton J S 1948 Simple ptosis operation: utilisation of frontalis muscle by means of a single rhomboid-shaped suture. Am J Ophthalmol 31: 411–414

Gaines R W Jr, Abernathie D L 1986 Mersilene tapes as a substitute for wire in segmental spinal instrumentation for children. Spine 11: 907–913

Giles G G, Marks R, Foley P 1988 Incidence of non-melanotic skin cancer treated in Australia. Br Med J 296: 13–17

Gladstein A H 1978 Radiotherapy of eyelid tumours. In: Jakobiec F A (ed) Ocular and adnexal tumours. Aesculapius, Birmingham

Gooding C A, White G, Yatsuhashi M 1965 Significance of marginal extension in excised basal cell carcinoma. N Engl J Med 273: 923–924

Hall V L, Leppard B J, McGill J et al 1986 Treatment of basal cell carcinoma: comparison of radiotherapy and cryotherapy. Clin Radiol 37: 33–34

Henderson J W 1965 Relief of eyelid retraction: a surgical procedure. Arch Ophthalmol 74: 205–216

Holt P J A 1988 Cryotherapy for skin cancer: results over a 5 year period using liquid nitrogen spray cryosurgery. Br J Dermatol 119: 231–240

Johnston R H Jr, Garcia-Rinaldi R, Vaugh G D et al 1985 Mersilene ribbon closure of the median sternotomy: an improvement over wire closure. Ann Thorac Surg 39: 88–89

Karesh J W, Fabrega M, Rodrigues M et al 1989 Polytetrafluoroethylene as an interpositional graft material for the correction of lower eyelid retraction. Ophthalmology 96: 419–423

Katowitz J A 1979 Frontalis suspension in congenital ptosis using a polyfilament cable type suture. Arch Ophthalmol 97: 1659–1663

Lisman R D, Smith B C 1987 Eyelid surgery for thyroid ophthalmopathy. In: Smith B C, Della Roca R C, Nesi F A et al (eds) Ophthalmic plastic and reconstructive surgery. Mosby, St Louis

Lubritz R R 1977 Cryosurgical management of the multiple skin carcinomas. J Derm Surg Oncol 3: 414–416

Mazur D 1970 Cryobiology: the freezing of biological systems. Science 168: 934–949

McIntosh G S, Li A K C, Osborne D R et al 1983 Basal cell carcinoma: a review of treatment results with special reference to cryotherapy. Postgrad Med J 59: 698–701

Mohs F E 1941 Chemosurgery, a microscopically controlled method of cancer excision. Arch Surg 42: 279–295

Mohs F E 1976 Chemosurgery for skin cancer: fixed and fresh tissue techniques. Arch Dermatol 112: 211–215

Mohs F E 1978 Chemosurgery: microscopically controlled surgery for skin cancer. Thomas, Springfield, IL

Neel H B, Ketcham A S, Hammond W G 1973 Experimental evaluation of in situ oncoside for primary tumour therapy: comparison of tumour specific immunity after complete excision cryonecrosis and ligation. Laryngoscope 83: 375–387

Nichols D A 1973 The Mersilene mesh gauze hammock for severe urinary stress incontinence. Obstet Gynecol 41: 88–93

Pusey W A 1907 The use of carbon dioxide snow in the treatment of naevi and other lesions of the skin. J Am Med Assoc 49: 1354–1356

Richards S, Brodstein R, Richards W et al 1988 Long-term course of surgically induced astigmatism. J Cataract Refractive Surg 14: 270–276

Rodriguez-Sains R S, Jakobiec F A 1987 Eyelid and conjunctival neoplasms. In: Smith B C, Della Roca R C, Nesi F A et al (eds) Ophthalmic plastic and reconstructive surgery. Mosby, St Louis

Shephard J 1979 The effect of low temperature on dermal connective tissue components. MSc thesis, University of Oxford

Shephard J, Dawber R P R 1982 The historical and scientific basis of cryosurgery. Clin Exp Dermatol 7: 321–328

Sirivella S, Zikria E A, Ford W B et al 1987 Improved technique for closure of median sternotomy incision. J Thorac Cardiovasc Surg 94: 591–595

Soanes W A, Gonder M J, Albin R J 1969 Clinical and experimental aspects of prostatic cryosurgery. J Cryosurg 2: 23–28

Tillett C W, Tillett G M 1966 Silicone sling in the correction of ptosis. Am J Ophthalmol 62: 521–523

Torre D 1971 Cryosurgery of pre-malignant and malignant skin lesions. Cutis 8: 123–129

Torre D 1977 Cryosurgical treatment of epitheliomas using the cone spray technique. J Dermatol Surg Oncol 3: 432–436

Tromovitch T A, Stegeman S J 1974 Microscopically controlled excision of skin tumours. Arch Dermatol 110: 231–232

Victorian Cancer Registry, Melbourne 1983. Skin cancer: an Australian health hazard

Waller R R, McCord C D Jr, Tanenbaum M 1987 Evaluation and management of the ptosis patient. In: McCord C D Jr, Tanenbaum M (eds) Oculoplastic surgery, 2nd edn. Raven Press, New York

White A C 1899 Liquid air in its application in medicine and surgery. Med Records 56: 109–112

Whitehouse H H 1907 Liquid air in dermatology: its indications and limitations. J Am Med Assoc 49: 371–377

Zacarian S A 1969 Cryosurgery for skin cancer and cryogenic techniques in dermatology. Thomas, Springfield, IL

Zacarian S A 1972 Cancer of the eyelid: a cryosurgical approach. Ann Ophthalmol 4: 473–480

Zacarian S A 1977 Cryosurgery for cancer of the skin. In: Cryosurgical advances in dermatology and tumours of the head and neck. Thomas, Springfield, II.

2

Contact lens practice

R. Buckley   J. Morris

INTRODUCTION

Contact lenses were first made in the 1880s. Glass was the material used until the 1930s, when PMMA (acrylic) became available, and made possible the micro-corneal lens. Soft hydrogel materials appeared in the 1970s and gas-permeable rigid materials soon afterwards. Recent developments have seen the emergence of materials that are much more compatible with the normal corneal physiology than was formerly possible. Contact lens-associated disease has been categorized and methodically investigated. The dangers of microbial keratitis, especially in connection with the continuous (extended) wear of soft lenses, have been assessed and remain the subject of basic and clinical research. Whilst the contact lens industry is currently feeling the effects of economic recession, contact lens science and medicine continue to expand at challenging speed. This chapter reviews some of the more significant recent developments in the field.

MATERIALS

Soft lenses

Soft lens materials and designs have proliferated since the early 1970s. In the early years the design of lenses, particularly with regard to their thickness, was the main point of concern; later their water content became of greater interest. The rationale for higher water content is to allow as much oxygen as possible to reach the cornea, especially at the limbus. The permeability (Dk) and transmissibility (Dk/t) give a measurement of oxygen flux through the material and lens to the cornea; but the equivalent oxygen percentage (EOP) profiles (Fig. 2.1) give a better idea of the potential problems of individual designs and back vertex powers, especially with regard to their performance at the limbus (Efron & Brennan 1987). The available atmospheric oxygen is 21%, reducing to 7.5% in sleep. The first signs of corneal oedema are seen at 10%. The profiles accurately indicate the overall lens/oxygen performance from centre to lens edge in relation to these conditions. This is particularly important for the closed eye situation when a soft lens is to be used for extended wear.

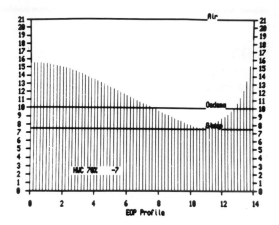

Fig. 2.1   Equivalent oxygen percentage (EOP) profile of a high-water-content lens, showing the effect of the lens edge thickness reducing oxygen availability to the limbal area. (Profile courtesy of K. H. Edwards.)

An ultra-thin high-water-content lens would be the theoretical ideal but at present this is impractical because the lens would be extremely fragile and, because of dehydration upon wearing, corneal desiccation would be a major problem (Zantos et al 1986). Dehydration is determined by the balance between free and bound water. Some materials incorporate methacrylic acid to help bind water more strongly (Hart 1987). These materials are known as ionic materials and have the potential of being less affected by dehydration, while those without this addition are known as non-ionic. However, the induced negative surface charge on ionic materials does cause greater deposition (Minarik & Rapp 1989) and there is also a potential for problems caused by pH changes and tonicity factors of the care regimens used. Hence, some non-ionic materials are claimed to be more deposit resistant than others, especially in the low (30–45%) and medium (50–65%) water content ranges, because the lower the water content the more resistant to deposition is the material.

The method of manufacture of soft hydrogel lenses has some bearing on their performance as it influences the surface produced. Smoother surfaces result from the original spin cast method and from the newer moulding methods, rather than from lathe cutting. The method of manufacture to some extent determines the reproducibility and ready availability of soft lenses.

As our knowledge of the oxygen requirements of the normal cornea has improved, it has become apparent that no hydrogel lens of any material, thickness or power is capable of providing the cornea with sufficient oxygen during sleep. This oxygen is necessary to prevent a greater than physiological overnight increase in thickness which would result from the hypoxia. Even for daily wear, the combination of water content, thickness and power must be carefully judged if the cornea is to receive its minimal open-eye oxygen requirement. From a practical point of view, even for daily wear, it has been found advisable that for powers over -4.00 dioptres a lens of at least 65% water content be fitted (Efron & Brennan 1987).

Deposition on the surface of soft lenses tends to be mainly due to protein, calcium and lipid constituents of the tears. Lipids are a major constituent of deposits and this problem can be accentuated by tear deficiency and occasionally diet (Hart et al 1986, 1987). As the surface of the material, its nature and the care regimen all have a part to play in the incidence of deposits, it is understandable that the current trend is towards more frequent replacement of lenses and towards disposable systems.

'Frequent-replacement systems' are now being promoted by a number of contact lens manufacturers based upon a selection of their lenses. The usual recommendation is a three- or six-monthly replacement programme. The regular replacement of the lens before ageing changes spoil its surface properties leads to fewer surface-related wearing problems; furthermore aftercare is encouraged as the patient needs to visit the practitioner before the issue of each new pair of lenses.

Disposable contact lenses

1988 was the year in which the first disposable contact lenses arrived in the UK and since then two other systems have been launched. They are all designed as extended-wear systems but can be used for daily wear. Because of the high incidence of corneal infection associated with the extended wear of contact lenses, this mode of wear cannot be condoned for cosmetic purposes. The lenses should be worn on a daily basis, cleaned and disinfected after wear and discarded either weekly or fortnightly. The choice of disposal interval is made by the practitioner on the basis of the rate of lens spoilation in the individual. Weekly and two-weekly disposal does seem to reduce such adverse reactions as acute epithelial necrosis due to tight lens syndrome, and papillary conjunctivitis (Grant & Holden 1988), but chronic hypoxia and contact lens-related infection are at the same level as for other daily-worn hydrogel lenses.

The disposable contact lens is a marketing concept rather than a distinct type of contact lens. It is a concept that appeals strongly to many wearers who, on the whole, are not prepared to comply with complex care routines. When such individuals are told that they must wear these lenses on a daily basis and furthermore must clean and disinfect them every day, the disposable concept becomes much less attractive and moreover the cost of solutions (in addition to the cost of the lenses) is a disincentive. The ideal disposable lens is the lens that is discarded at the end of each day. At present, the cost would be prohibitive for all but the most affluent wearer, but it is possible that improvements in manufacture and in packaging will allow this goal to be realized.

Most of the disposable lenses currently available are of the 'one-fit' variety and so not every patient can be fitted. As yet there are no complex designs available, such as torics or bifocals. It is obviously not feasible for the practitioner to check each lens before it is worn and so one is reliant on the reproducibility of the manufacture and the availability of a bank of lenses from which to supply the patient as necessary. The exercise of retailing disposable contact lenses involves the practitioner in a complex administrative system.

Possibly the only medical indication for disposable contact lenses is lens-related papillary conjunctivitis. Early on in the history of this condition it was observed by patients and practitioners that new lenses relieve both symptoms and signs for a short time.

Rigid gas-permeable lenses

Contact lenses have come nearly full circle from the advent in 1938 of polymethylmethacrylate (PMMA) as a suitable contact lens material. After the years of soft lens fitting with its early promise to some wearers, but the later-perceived disadvantages to others from the short and long-term effects, the advent of the rigid gas-permeable lens was welcomed by contact lens practitioners. The oxygen permeability of the newer materials has now risen beyond soft lens capabilities, thanks to the efforts of polymer chemists who have created cocktails of PMMA, cellulose acetate butyrate and silicone. The silicone acrylates have been the major constituent materials until recently, when the element fluorine entered the contact lens field.

Fluorine is usually formulated with siloxane-acrylate or vinyl pyrrolidone-methyl methacrylate to give high oxygen transmissibility, good wetting, a deposit-resistant surface and good tensile strength. These excellent properties do not, however, preclude trouble in the clinical environment. The problems can start at the manufacturing stage where polymerization has not been uniform and lenses may then suffer from increased brittleness and surface defects. After a few months of wear, surface cracking and crazing occur (Walker 1990), which with fluorosilicone acrylates may be only 1 μm in depth, but the consequences of microbial colonization of these altered surfaces do cause concern (Grohe et al 1987). Mucus coats these lenses, as with all others, and there may be the same wetting problems as are found in any of the other hard gas-permeable lenses; inevitably protein deposition occurs in some patients (Fatt 1985). Even so, contact lens-induced papillary conjunctivitis does seem to be reduced with these lenses, if worn on an extended-wear basis, compared with soft lenses (Holden & Sweeney 1987). Fluoropolymers are physically rather flexible and this can cause visual problems, especially in astigmatic eyes, unless they are fitted for minimal flexure (Stone & Collins 1984, Stevenson & Cornish 1990). However, the oxygen transmissibility is sufficient to allow these lenses to be worn on an extended-wear basis (Schnider et al 1987) and it appears that the level of oxygen at the corneal surface is adequate to avoid significant epithelial compromise in the majority of patients (Holden & Sweeney 1987).

Others

Silicone elastomer

This has been used for contact lenses since 1962 but has never progressed beyond the description 'the material of the future'. It is a highly oxygen-permeable material with excellent optical qualities, is quite flexible, very resilient and chemically and physiologically inert. However, it does have the major problem of surface hydrophobicity and the lenses tend to bind to the cornea (Roth et al 1980). As lens movement and tear exchange is vital to corneal health the binding property of the silicone lens has virtually removed it from the cosmetic market. It is now fitted only for specific medical indications, for example as a therapeutic lens, where there is a reasonable measure of success (Woodward 1984).

Collagen

Reconstituted from a porcine source, collagen has been used to manufacture therapeutic contact lenses which gradually dissolve in the tear film and additionally serve to increase the contact time of drops concurrently applied. When fully hydrated, these lenses have a high water content (around 90%) and a moderate oxygen transmissibility. Comfort and wetting are generally good. As yet, collagen has not been successfully used in the cosmetic market, but it is seen as having a possible future role as a disposable lens.

The ideal contact lens material has yet to be discovered but the qualities it needs are known: high oxygen permeability, good wetting characteristics, resistance to deposition, strength, dimensional stability and reproducibility. A mixture of HEMA (hydroxyethyl-methacrylate), silicone and hard gas-permeable constituents should be favourable for all of those needs — a 'hard/soft' material, possibly. Until now the only lens to appear which could perhaps eventually fill all of these parameters is a hard gas-permeable material with a copolymerized hydrophilic periphery. Unfortunately the manufacture of this hybrid lens continues to pose problems and it has been only intermittently available. It has just been relaunched by Pilkington Barnes-Hind as the 'SoftPerm' lens

DESIGN

The design of hard and soft lenses has expanded over the years and now even soft materials can be made into toric and bifocal lenses. Spherical lenses in soft materials are monocurve or bicurve and it is postulated that bicurves decentre less (Young 1990).

Aspheric lenses

Also now available are back and front aspheric designs which can help in lens centration (Forst 1984) or can be design manipulated to reduce the thickness of the lens in high powers (Bleshoy 1985). Visually, a reduction in spherical aberration has been reported (Kerns 1974) while early presbyopes may be helped with their near vision (Mayers 1983). Rigid gas-permeable aspheric lenses are also available as many corneal models are now hypothesized (Bibby 1976, Kiely et al 1984, Guillon et al 1986). Although these aspheric lenses do have a small spherical edge to aid tear exchange, the conformity of fit helps to spread evenly the weight of the lens on the cornea.

Toric lenses

Advances in toric designs and their methods of stabilization have enabled more of the astigmatic population to be fitted with soft lenses in recent years. The truncated lens has proved less popular because of problems associated with the straight edge but prism-ballasted lenses are now available in a number of designs. The other two main methods of stabilization are by chamfering the top and bottom edges so that the thin portions fit under the lids (Grant 1986) and by lens elevations or orientation cams (Freitag 1989). All of these designs can be manufactured in various water content materials and although vision is often compromised by fluctuations caused by movement, many more patients are now successful toric lens wearers than were previously.

Hard toric designs have changed little except that materials of high permeability can be used. Some aspheric/spherical designs, because of their close conformity to the corneal shape, can correct up to 4 dioptres of corneal astigmatism in some patients; this is an easier option than fitting a toric lens with its problems of stabilization and induced astigmatism. The flexure of spherical hard gas-permeable lenses can also be used to deal with corneal astigmatism. By fitting flatter, the residual astigmatism is reduced because of the minimal flexure (Stone & Collins 1984) and so in some cases a spherical lens can be fitted rather than a toric design.

Bifocal lenses

The popularity of contact lenses over the years has meant that there is now a large group of presbyopic patients who are not used to wearing spectacles. The usual type of patient asking for bifocal contact lenses is the long-term wearer, but even more non-wearers are also now aware of the availability of bifocal contact lenses. However, one of the main contraindications to bifocal lens wear is the patient with a refraction in the plano to low hypermetropic range whose distance vision will inevitably be compromised by a bifocal design.

PMMA, rigid gas-permeable and soft lens bifocals are all available. The designs are either 'alternating' or 'simultaneous' vision. The alternating-vision bifocals work on the principle of the patient either viewing a distance or a near object which comes into view by either the straight ahead or the downward gaze of the eyes, vertical translation of the lens being achieved by contact with the lower lid margin. Simultaneous vision is where the desired in-focus image of the distance or near object is always accompanied by a superimposed out-of-focus image formed by the remainder of the correction (Charman & Saunders 1990).

In the rigid gas-permeable materials a new alternating design and different simultaneous designs are now available. The alternating bifocal named the Tangent Streak is of monocentric design and works on the principle of the executive spectacle bifocal. As with all alternating designs, it needs support from the lower lid to translate. It differs from other alternating designs in the size of the reading area, which is much larger than the usual fused or solid segments. The lens is also fitted to allow more movement than normal to help it translate; this can be counterproductive because of excessive cyclorotation (Josephson & Caffrey 1989).

Most bifocals are influenced in their effectiveness by variations in pupil diameter. However, a non-pupil-dependent diffractive bifocal has been designed by Freeman & Stone (1987) and is marketed as the Diffrax by Pilkington Barnes-Hind (Fig. 2.2). A circular phase plate is incorporated into the lens optic. Light is made to interfere constructively at two focal points, and to interfere destructively at other points on the optic axis. Although the advantage of clear near vision in all directions of gaze should be available with this design there is a general loss of image contrast (Charman & Saunders 1990). A soft lens diffractive bifocal by Allergan Optical, the Echelon, has diffracting facets ('Echelettes') that are a large number of Fresnel-type reading zones. This design also suffers from a decrease in contrast of the retinal image (Papas et al 1989).

Aspheric surfaces are used in soft lens bifocals to provide progressive addition lenses. Back-surface aspherics are designed with the power in the

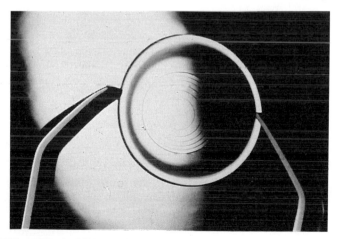

Fig. 2.2 Diffrax bifocal. (Pilkington Barnes-Hind.)

centre correct for distance, while the periphery provides the near addition (Bausch & Lomb PA1 and Hydrocurve II by Pilkington Barnes-Hind). The greater the eccentricity, the higher the near addition, and the greater the range over which objects are in focus. However, the greater the pupil diameter, the larger is the fall in image contrast (Charman & Walsh 1988). Front surface aspherics (Nissel PS 45 and the Unilens) are designed such that the power becomes progressively less positive towards the lens periphery in a centre-near design which is therefore not compromised by constriction of the pupil on close work. Charman & Saunders (1988) have found that there is a variation in addition across the range of distance powers, so changes in pupil diameter are likely to affect performance.

Monovision

The visual compromises still presented by today's bifocal contact lenses have meant that some patients seek a different option. Fitting the non-dominant eye with a lens for near vision while leaving the dominant eye corrected for distance is often a successful means of dealing with the presbyopic patient (Back et al 1987). One of the main drawbacks to this method is the resulting loss of stereopsis (Heath et al 1986) which might have legal significance should the patient be involved in an accident of some kind (Harris & Classe 1988). Often a third lens can be supplied to be worn for prolonged driving. 'Monovision' can also be achieved with a centre-near bifocal in the non-dominant eye. Myopic patients may have slipped into monovision with their current single vision lenses because of refractive changes and so become ideal candidates for this simple method of presbyopic correction.

Success in bifocal contact lens fitting is increased if one has a selection of lenses available and also if a combination of designs is tried (Table 2.1).

Table 2.1

Dominant eye	Non-dominant eye
Distance single vision	Centre-near bifocal
Centre-distance bifocal	Centre-near bifocal
Centre-distance bifocal	Near single vision
Distance single vision	Near single vision

CARE REGIMENS

The care of both soft and rigid gas-permeable lenses has been and continues to be a problem for both the patient and the practitioner. The patient often finds the multiplicity of steps needed and the cost involved to be deterrents, while the practitioner calls for effective cleaning and disinfecting solutions that are not toxic to the cornea and are physically compatible with the lens material.

In the UK each solution goes through regulatory control by the Department of Health. Data have to be submitted that satisfies the DOH Committees on the quality, safety and efficacy of the solution. Nevertheless, over the years it has become apparent that long-term use under actual clinical conditions can give rise to unforeseen problems. The practitioner must therefore explain the principles of cleaning and disinfection in terms suitable for the understanding of each patient. He must satisfy himself that each patient continues to use the appropriate solutions effectively. Careful, detailed questioning is usually necessary, as solution misuse is one of the biggest aftercare problems (Collins & Carney 1986, Chun & Weissman 1987) and a significant cause of the corneal infections seen in contact lens practice today (Barry & Ruben 1980, Mathews et al 1983).

Soft lenses

The disinfection of soft lenses falls into two categories: heat and chemical. Heat disinfection with unpreserved saline (from a single-use sachet or a pressure canister) is still an effective method of controlling the organisms present on the lens but it can denature protein on the hydrophilic surface, which then becomes a cumulative problem. It also discolours high-water-content materials and so if heat disinfection is used such lenses will need frequent replacement.

Chemical disinfection has moved away from preserved systems because of the well-documented effects of preservatives such as thiomersal being retained in the polymer matrix and then leaching out of the lenses in wear, so causing a sensitivity reaction (Wilson 1980, Wright & Mackie 1982). A new preparation providing 0.004% chlorhexidine gluconate has recently been introduced in a uniquely formulated tablet (OptimEyes). The storage medium is potable tap water available from rising mains and experimentally the preparation shows good antimicrobial activity (Davies et al 1988). Patient compliance with such a simple system is expected to be good. The product is currently being marketed along with a disposable soft contact lens.

Chemical disinfection of soft contact lenses is either by hydrogen peroxide or by a chlorine releasing agent. The chlorine based systems contain either sodium dichloroisocyanurate (Softab) or para-dichlorosulphamyl benzoic acid (Acrotab). These are also one-step systems to help compliance, but residual traces of the active disinfecting agents may be present on lens insertion, and furthermore it has been found that the chlorine-based systems have poor anti-Acanthamoeba activity (Meakin 1989).

Hydrogen peroxide systems are usually based on a 3% solution. All have sodium or phosphate stabilizers because peroxide is unstable and rapidly decomposes. The systems available in the UK are all two-step methods and are either catalytic or reactive. The catalytic method uses catalase, a naturally occurring bovine catalyst which is highly specific for fast decomposition (Oxysept) or a platinum-coated disc that acts as a catalyst for the decomposition of hydrogen peroxide (Septicon). The reactive methods use a chemical to initiate an oxidation–reduction reaction for decomposition. The chemicals used are sodium pyruvate (Ciba Vision 10 : 10) and sodium thiosulphate (Perform). By-products such as bicarbonate and sulphates are formed with these systems.

The systems were originally intended to be used with a short soak of the lenses in the peroxide solution (e.g. 10 minutes) and a long overnight soak in the neutralizer. This was advised because soft contact lens parameters and water content can be influenced during hydrogen peroxide disinfection by pH and tonicity changes (Janoff 1985, Bruce 1989). The lens is, however, then left in an unsterile medium overnight. Recent work on antimicrobial kill curves (Meakin 1989) shows that overnight storage in the peroxide solution is a preferable time for complete deactivation. Yet the parameters of ionic high-water-content lenses are especially affected by this system and need time to regain their original shape (McKenney 1990).

Cleaning fluids used with manual application nightly are vital for lens care. The routine should be carried out on removal of the lens from the eye and before disinfection. The removal of contaminants such as lipids, some proteins and inorganic deposits enhances the antibacterial activity of the disinfectant. Solutions preserved with thiomersal, chlorhexidine or sorbic acid (LC65, Bausch & Lomb, Pliagel) can be used with all soft lenses but those preserved with benzalkonium chloride must not be used, because of its property of binding to the hydrophilic matrix (Clens, Transclean, Hydron). The main unpreserved cleaning solution available uses isopropyl alcohol (Mira-flow) which has good anti-*Acanthamoeba* activity and so should be used in conjunction with those disinfection systems whose activity is low (Penley et al 1989).

Protein removal tablets are used by most patients on a prophylactic basis between weekly and monthly depending on the practitioner's assessment of the need. They are used dissolved in sterile saline and now faster-action tablets are available which for soft lenses require only a 15-minute soak. Tablets which deal with protein, lipids and mucin are available, the active ingredients being papain, pancreatin or protease with lipase and pronase. A system using such tablets in the peroxide solution is now available; the active ingredient is subtilisin A (Ultrazyme). Rewetting or comfort drops, if resorted to, tend to indicate poor contact lens tolerance. They are of course necessary in patients who have a tear deficiency. Unpreserved saline (Clerz) is the most useful aid to lens hydration.

Disinfection of the practitioner's trial soft lenses is important not only because of ordinary cross-infection hazards but also because the HIV agent has been isolated in the tear fluid (Fujikawa et al 1986). As yet contact lenses have not been proven to transmit the HIV agent from one individual to another but the potential exists. All current methods of disinfection kill the HIV organism but heat disinfection is the most reliable. If heat is normally used, however, one will have to change the trial lenses more frequently.

Hard gas-permeable lenses

The use of preservatives in contact lens solutions for gas-permeable lenses is much less of a problem than for soft lenses as the solutions do not enter the material. However, there has been a controversy surrounding the use of benzalkonium chloride (BAK) with gas-permeable lenses for the last ten years (Hoffman 1987). There have been instances where BAK has been reported to reduce the lens wettability (Rosenthal et al 1986), whereas other reports show no difference in action on the surface to the PMMA material for which it has been used for many years (Walters et al 1983). Therefore, there is a multitude of solutions containing all acceptable preservatives for the soaking, wetting and cleaning of gas-permeable lenses.

A cleaning solution containing polymeric beads (which tend to have a polishing action on the lens surface) is useful for patients who deposit heavily on their lenses (Bausch & Lomb, Boston). This preparation, and its companion soaking and wetting solution, is preserved with chlorhexidine. Protein removal tablets often have to be used with gas-permeable lenses and soaking is for two or more hours. Rewetting drops, which are usually in the form of artificial tears, are sometimes necessary, but their routine use should not be condoned.

COMPLICATIONS

In a recent case-controlled study from the Accident and Emergency Department of Moorfields Eye Hospital, estimates were made of the relative risks of different contact lens types for five groups of complications (Stapleton et al 1989a, Dart 1991). The groups of complications were metabolic, abrasive, toxic and hypersensitivity responses, infections and sterile corneal infiltrates. The relative risks, compared to hard gas-permeable lenses, were 20.8 times for extended-wear soft lenses, 3.6 times for daily-wear soft lenses and 1.2 times for PMMA wearers. These trends were significant.

PMMA

Contact lenses made of PMMA have now been worn for as long as 30 years. The most serious long-term effect of this material is chronic hypoxia, which results in patients showing a corneal sensitivity reduction of a factor of 2 (Millodot 1978). Morphological changes to the endothelium (MacRae et al 1985), which are virtually irreversible and which, it has been suggested, place the cornea at greater risk from surgery, are also important long-term effects (Rao et al 1979). Hypoxic corneal stress also gives rise to corneal warpage, which is difficult to manage clinically. These patients can often be refitted with high-oxygen gas-permeable materials with a consequent return of a degree of corneal sensitivity and a decrease in warpage. Many long-standing PMMA wearers have chronic horizontal peripheral drying ('three and nine o'clock staining') which results in vascularized areas of opaque tissue.

However, PMMA is a robust, easy to maintain and stable material which does not always produce unacceptable changes during wear so there are many patients who may be continued in this material with competent annual monitoring.

Soft lenses

The complications of daily-wear soft lenses are mostly hypoxia related or due to the misuse of solutions. The limbal vessels of most long-term soft lens wearers show congestion or elongation, but it is the new deep stromal vessels whose appearance warrants immediate abandonment of soft lens wear in cosmetic cases, due to the added possibility of lipid deposition in the adjacent tissue. The low-water-content lenses worn on an all-day basis also show myopic creep (Grosvenor 1975) and endothelial cell morphological changes (MacRae et al 1986), so low-water lenses should only be used in ultra-thin designs (e.g. 0.07 mm or less), otherwise medium to high-water-content lenses should be fitted.

Hygiene

Lens hygiene is an increasing problem in contact-lens-wearing patients, as was first shown at Moorfields Eye Hospital in the study by Barry & Ruben (1980), where in 217 contact lens casualties over half had storage cases which were contaminated with bacteria. Poor lens hygiene is now strongly associated with contact-lens-related infiltrates (Stapleton et al 1989b) as is the type of lens being worn. Stapleton and her colleagues (1989b) found that the risk of sterile infiltrates was significantly higher for extended soft lens wearers compared with gas-permeable lens wearers at 2.33 times, while it was 1.56 times with daily-wear soft lenses, and lowest with PMMA wearers at 0.51 times. Microbial infection may follow either adherence of the bacteria to the lens material or the secretion by the bacterium of its own polysaccharide biofilm, either of which can result in the creation of a massive potential bacterial inoculum. Then an epithelial breach may present a favourable environment for bacterial invasion (Dart et al 1988). This breach is easily achieved in contact lens wearers, especially in those people wearing lenses on an extended-wear basis, as they show a reduction in epithelial adhesion (Madigan & Holden 1988). The use of disposable soft lenses also carries this risk factor for the patient (Parker & Wong 1989). As *Pseudomonas aeruginosa* is a virulent corneal pathogen to which the contact lens patient is particularly predisposed, especially those wearing soft lenses (Dart 1987), is it always important to isolate the pathogen in the lens wearer before deciding to patch an apparently innocent 'contact lens abrasion'.

Keratitis due to *Acanthamoeba polyphaga* or *A. castellani* has been reported usually in daily-wear soft lens (Moore et al 1987). While home-made saline has been implicated as one source of contamination (Ficker 1988) a study has been carried out in which the home environment of 43 asymptomatic and 6 recently infected contact lens wearers was inspected. Stapleton and colleagues (1990) isolated *Acanthamoeba* sp. from 6 bathroom cold water samples (5 with scale), 1 kitchen cold water sample, 1 bathroom dust sample and 2 bathroom drains. Thirty per cent of the patients rinsed their cases in bathroom tap water before cleaning and disinfection. It is advisable to recommend rinsing the case thoroughly with boiled water and then allowing it to dry in air.

The tarsal plate

All contact lens wearers show upper tarsal plate changes due to the mechanical aspect of lens wear. Contact-lens-induced papillary conjunctivitis is more frequently seen in atopes, in patients wearing lenses coated with proteins and in those using preserved care systems or heat disinfection. Soft lenses coat more readily than hard gas-permeable materials, which coat more than PMMA, but the trigger mechanism can be the type of protein rather than the amount (Grant et al 1989). Cleaning cannot be totally effective in removing all of the coating material, especially from soft lenses, and this is one reason why disposable soft lenses have recently been marketed. Once the patient has irritation and mucous discharge, the condition is advanced and must be treated. Contact lens wear can be discontinued, or the material and care system changed with frequent replacements of the lenses if of a hydrophilic type. Disodium cromoglycate drops and ointment are most satisfactory with atopic individuals, while topical steroid can be tried in intractable cases, provided that they remain under regular ophthalmological supervision.

THERAPEUTIC CONTACT LENSES

Recent advances in therapeutic contact lens work have involved the use of different materials and their use in solving recognized problems. As new materials become available in contact lens practice their application in therapeutic fitting is always studied.

Soft and silicone lenses

Soft lenses in plano power varying from low- to high-water content have been used for many years as therapeutic lenses, particularly to reduce pain or facilitate healing. However, an eye with significant tear deficiency which allows the rapid drying of a soft lens, making it impossible to wear, can now be fitted with a silicone rubber lens. The hydrophobic nature of the silicone material allows it to retain its physical properties on dry eyes and to deal with exposure problems following lid reconstruction. Furthermore, because of its defined shape, it can be useful on perforated corneae to avoid surgery while allowing time for healing (Woodward 1984). Silicone rubber has been used for many years in infantile and elderly aphakic eyes on both an extended and a daily-wear basis, with reasonable success.

Hard gas-permeable lenses

Hard gas-permeable materials with their higher oxygen transmission have been successful in keratoconus designs and in fitting other corneal irregularities. They are the material of first choice for eyes after radial keratotomy, when PMMA is best avoided because of possible corneal oedema and warpage, while soft lenses can give rise to vascularization and there is also a risk of infection (Astin 1986). Post-radial keratotomy eyes are difficult to fit as the cornea's shape factor changes from positive towards negative, so that it has a flat centre with a steep periphery, the converse of normal.

Scleral lenses

Scleral lens wearers may also benefit from hard gas-permeable materials, and preformed lenses made of these materials have been described (Ezekiel 1983). The manufacture of lenses from an eye impression is complicated as hard gas-permeable materials are not readily available in sheet form and are not suitably thermolabile (Pullum 1987). The brittleness of the material and the wettability of the surface have caused further problems in manufacturing and wear. Patients did, however, find hard gas-permeable (HGP) scleral lenses more comfortable than their own PMMA lenses in a pilot study carried out at Moorfields Eye Hospital (Pullum et al 1989). Further work has been done to investigate the corneal thickening associated with HGP scleral lens wear, especially as the thickness of the lenses is an important factor in the risk of breakage as well as in the transmission of oxygen. Pullum and colleagues (1990) investigated two gas-permeable lens materials of low and high oxygen permeability against PMMA made in a sealed scleral design. The results did show a smaller increase in central corneal thickening between the gas-permeable materials and the PMMA lens over 3 hours of wear (Table 2.2) and confirmed the results of earlier work by Bleshoy & Pullum (1988), which showed that lenses of varying thicknesses up to 0.60 mm did not produce entirely predictable degrees of corneal swelling.

Cosmetic lenses

To cover unsightly corneae soft lenses are available, while other cases are best dealt with by a rigid cosmetic shell. Soft lens tinting has improved over recent years and now the matching of the other, normal, eye is much more successful. Transparent or opaque tints are available with or without black pupils. Total occlusion for patching young children is still difficult to achieve by contact lenses, but these lenses do have a place in the management of

Table 2.2 Percentage increase in central corneal thickening recorded for both subjects wearing scleral lenses of varying materials and thicknesses

Scleral lens material and thickness (mm)	% increase in CCT of the test eye			
	Subject 1 (1 SD)		Subject 2 (1 SD)	
PMMA	9.59	0.16	11.24	0.67
24 Dk (1.2)			11.29	0.35
(0.6)	6.07	0.76	6.92	0.61
(0.3)	7.60	0.00	5.34	1.73
(0.15)	3.50	1.85	5.19	1.53
115 Dk (1.2)			5.47	2.00
(0.6)	2.00	1.56	1.68	0.47
(0.3)	1.29	0.47	1.84	0.58
(0.15)	0.73	0.76	2.88	0.67

Reproduced with kind permission of the *Journal of the British Contact Lens Association.*

intractable diplopia. However, as in all contact lens wear, the eye has to be able to tolerate a lens and the underlying tissue should not interfere with the lens fitting.

Children

Infants and children continue to benefit from contact lens wear for aphakia and high myopia. The unilateral cases are less successful and where a hard gas-permeable lens is indicated for optical reasons this can often be difficult for the child to tolerate when only one eye is involved.

CONCLUSION

As we approach the year 2000 contact lens practice will continue to expand through the development of new materials and designs. Both the abnormal and the normal eye will benefit from the research being conducted, both by manufacturers and in scientific and medical institutions. The ideal contact lens does not yet exist, but unfortunately the complications that arise from this foreign body are as much patient determined as product associated.

REFERENCES

Astin C 1986 Contact lenses for patients after radial keratotomy. Trans Br Contact Lens Assoc Ann Clin Conf 3: 2–7
Back A P, Woods R, Holden B A 1987 The comparative visual performance of monovision and various concentric bifocals. Trans Br Contact Lens Assoc Ann Clin Conf 4: 46–47
Barry P J, Ruben M 1980 Contact lens injuries: analysis of 217 consecutive patients presenting to Moorfields casualty department. Contact Lens J 9: 6–10
Bibby M M 1976 Computer assisted photokeratoscopy and contact lens design. Optician 171:

37–43, 11–17, 15–17

Bleshoy H 1985 Aspheric aphakic soft lens design: clinical results. Contact Lens J 13: 11

Bleshoy H, Pullum K W 1988 Corneal response to gas permeable impression scleral lenses. J Br Contact Lens Assoc 1: 31–34

Brennen N A, Efron N 1989 Strategies for increasing the oxygen performance of hydrogel contact lenses. Contax (July): 12–18

Bruce A 1989 Hydration of hydrogel contact lenses during hydrogen peroxide disinfection. J Am Ophthalmol Assoc 60: 581–582

Charman W N, Saunders B 1988 Optical properties and patient acceptance of the Nissel PS45 presbyopic lens: a preliminary study. Optom Today (Feb 13): 100–106

Charman W N, Saunders B 1990 Theoretical and practical factors influencing the optical performance of contact lenses for the presbyope. J Br Contact Lens Assoc 13: 67–75

Charman W N, Walsh G 1988 Retinal images with centred, aspheric, varifocal contact lenses. Int Contact Lens Clin 13: 87–94

Chun M W, Weissman B A 1987 Compliance in contact lens care. Am J Optom Physiol Opt 64: 274–276

Collins M J, Carney L G 1986 Patient compliance and its influence on contact lens wearing problems. Am J Optom Physiol Opt 63: 952–956

Dart J K G 1987 Bacterial keratitis in contact lens users. Br Med J 295: 959–960

Dart J K G, Peacock J, Grierson I, Seal D V 1988 Ocular surface, contact lens and bacterial interactions in a rabbit model. Trans Br Contact Lens Assoc Int Cont Lens Centenary Cong 5: 95–97

Dart J K G 1991 Contact lens-associated infections. Proceedings of the 5th Workshop on Ext Eye Dis and Inflammation, Fisonsplc

Davies D J G, Anthony Y, Meakin B J et al 1988 Anti-Acanthamoeba activity of chlorhexidine and hydrogen peroxide. Trans Br Contact Lens Assoc Int Contact Lens Centenary Cong 5: 60–62

Efron N, Brennan N A 1987 In search of the critical oxygen requirement of the cornea. Contax (July): 5–11

Ezekiel D 1983 Gas permeable haptic lenses. J Br Contact Lens Assoc 6: 158–161

Fatt I 1985 A new look at fluoropolymers. Optician 190: 25–26

Ficker L 1988 Acanthamoeba keratitis: the quest for a better prognosis. Eye 2 (suppl): S37–S45

Forst G 1984 Aspheric contact lenses. Int Contact Lens Clin 12: 93–102

Freeman M H, Stone J 1987 A new diffractive bifocal contact lens. Trans Br Contact Lens Assoc Ann Clin Conf 1987: 15–22

Freitag C 1989 Clinical report on the Lunelle Toric Rx lens. Optom Today (Jan 28): 42–43

Fujikawa L S, Salahuddin S Z, Ablashi D 1986 HTLV III in the tears of AIDS patients. Ophthalmology 93: 1479–1481

Grant R 1986 The orientation of toric soft lenses. Contax (September): 8–10

Grant T, Holden B A 1988 The clinical performance of disposable (58%) extended wear lenses. Trans Br Contact Lens Assoc Int Cont Lens Centenary Cong 1988: 63–64

Grant T, Holden B A, Rechberger J, Chong M S 1989 Contact lens related papillary conjunctivitis (CLPC): influence of protein accumulation and replacement frequency. Invest Ophthalmol Vis Sci 30 (suppl): 166

Grohe R M, Caroline P J, Norman C et al 1987 Part II: Rigid gas permeable surface cracking: microbial concerns. Contact Lens Spectrum 2: 40–46

Grosvenor T 1975 Changes in corneal curvature and subjective refraction in soft contact lens wearers. Am J Optom Physiol Opt 52: 406–413

Guillon M, Lydon D P M, Wilson C 1986 Corneal topography: a clinical model. Ophthalmic Physiol Opt 6: 47–56

Harris M G, Classe J G 1988 Clinicolegal considerations of monovision. J Am Optom Assoc. 59: 491–495

Hart D E 1987 Surface interactions on hydrogel contact lenses: scanning electron microscopy

(SEM). J Am Optom Assoc 58: 962–974

Hart D E, Tisdale R R, Sack R A 1986 Origin and composition of lipid deposits on soft contact lenses. Ophthalmology 93: 495–503

Hart D E, Lane B C, Josephson J E et al 1987 Spoilage of hydrogel lenses by lipid deposits. Ophthalmology 94: 1315–1321

Heath D A, Hines C, Schwartz F 1986 Suppression behaviour analyzed as a function of monovision add power. Am J Optom 63: 198–201

Hoffman W C 1987 Ending the BAK–RGP controversy. Optician 193: 31–32

Holden B A, Sweeney D F 1987 Ocular requirements for extended wear. Contax (May): 13–18

Janoff L 1985 The exposure of various polymers to a 24-hour soak in Lensept: the effect on base curve. J Am Ophthalmol Assoc 56: 222–225

Josephson J E, Caffrey B E 1989 Clinical experience with the Tangent Streak RGP bifocal contact lens. J Am Optom Assoc 60: 166 170

Kerns R L 1974 Clinical evaluation of the merits of an aspheric front surface contact lens for patients manifesting residual astigmatism. Am J Optom Physiol Opt 51: 750–757

Kiely P M, Smith G, Carney L C 1984 Meridional variations in corneal shape. Am J Optom Physiol Opt 61: 619–626

MacRae S M, Matsuda M, Yee R 1985 The effect of long-term hard contact lens wear on the corneal endothelium. CLAO J 11: 322–326

MacRae S M, Matsuda M, Shellans S, Rich L F 1986 The effects of hard and soft contact lenses on the corneal endothelium. Am J Ophthalmol 102: 50–57

Madigan M C, Holden B A 1988 Factors involved in loss of epithelial adhesion (EA) with long-term continuous hydrogel lens wear. Invest Ophthalmol Vis Sci 29 (suppl): 253

Mathews A M, Dart J K G, Sherwood M 1983 Contact lens casualties: contact lens hygiene and related disease. J Br Contact Lens Assoc 6: 36–40

Mayers H B 1983 A clinical investigation of the CALS anterior surface aspheric hydrogel contact lens in the treatment of presbyopia. Can J Optom 45 (suppl): 8–13

McKenney C 1990 The effect of pH on hydrogel lens parameters and fitting characteristics after hydrogen peroxide disinfection. Trans Br Contact Lens Assoc Ann Clin Conf 46–51

Meakin B J 1989 Contact lens care systems: an update. Br Contact Lens Assoc Sci Meetings 26–31

Millodot M 1978 Effect of long-term wear of hard contact lenses on corneal sensitivity. Arch Ophthalmol 96: 1225–1227

Minarik L, Rapp J 1989 Protein deposits on individual hydrophilic contact lenses: effects of water and ionicity. CLAO J 15: 185–188

Moore M B, McCulley J P, Newton C et al 1987 Acanthamoeba keratitis: a growing problem in soft and hard contact lens wearers. Ophthalmology 94: 1654–1661

Papas E B, Young G, Hearn K 1989 Monovision versus diffractive bifocals. Trans Br Contact Lens Assoc Ann Clin Conf 75–76

Parker W T, Wong S K 1989 Keratitis associated with disposable soft contact lenses. Am J Ophthalmol 107: 195

Penley C A, Willis S W, Sickler S G 1989 Comparative antimicrobial efficacy of soft and rigid gas permeable contact lens solutions against Acanthamoeba. CLAO J 15: 257–260

Pullum K W 1987 Feasibility study for the production of gas permeable lenses using ocular impression techniques. Trans Br Contact Lens Assoc Ann Clin Conf 10: 35–39

Pullum K W, Parker J H, Hobley A J 1989 The Josef Dallos Award lecture 1989: development of gas permeable scleral lenses produced from impressions of the eye. Trans Br Contact Lens Assoc Ann Clin Conf 6: 77–81

Pullum K W, Hobley A J, Parker J H 1990 Hypoxic corneal changes following sealed gas permeable impression scleral lens wear. J Br Contact Lens Assoc 13: 83–87

Rao G N, Shaw E L, Arthur E J, Aquavella J V 1979 Endothelial cell morphology and corneal deturgescence. Ann Ophthalmol 11: 885–899

Rosenthal P, Chou M H, Salamone J C, Israel S C 1986 Quantitative analysis of chlorhexidine gluconate and benzalkonium chloride absorption of silicone/acrylate polymers. CLAO J 12: 43–50

Roth H W, Iwasaki W, Takayama M, Wada C 1980 Complication caused by silicon elastomer lenses in West Germany and Japan. Contact 24: 28–36

Schnider C, Holden B A, Terry R et al 1987 One and two year results from large scale clinical studies of RGP EW lenses. Invest Ophthalmol Vis Sci (suppl) 28: 372

Stapleton F, Dart J K G, Minassian D 1989a The relative risks of different contact lenses. ARVO (Suppl to Invest Ophthalmol Vis Sci) 12: 166

Stapleton F, Dart J K G, Minassian D 1989b Contact lens related infiltrates: risk figures for different lens types and association with lens hygiene and solution contamination. Trans Br Contact Lens Assoc Ann Clin Conf 6: 52–55

Stapleton F, Dart J K G, Seal D, Minassian D 1990 Possible sources of bacterial contamination in contact lens wearers with microbial keratitis. ARVO (suppl to Invest Ophthalmol Vis Sci) 883: 179

Stevenson R R W, Cornish R 1990 Fluorescein fitting patterns of RGP lenses: a clinical note. Optician 199: 31

Stone J, Collins C 1984 Flexure of gas permeable lenses on toroidal corneas. Optician 188: 8–10

Walker J 1990 Cracking and crazing: a practitioner's viewpoint. Optician 199: 19–21

Walters K, Gee H J, Meakin B J 1983 The interaction of benzalkonium chloride with Boston contact lens materials. J Br Contact Lens Assoc 6: 42–52

Wilson L A 1980 Thiomersal hypersensitivity in soft contact lens wearers. Contact Lens J 9: 21–24

Woodward E G 1984 Therapeutic silicone rubber lenses. J Br Contact Lens Assoc 7: 39–40

Wright P, Mackie I A 1982 Presevative-related problems in soft contact lens wearers. Trans Ophthalmol Soc UK 102: 3–6

Young G 1990 Design factors influencing contact lens performance. Paper given at Br Contact Lens Assoc Ann Clin Conf

Zantos S G, Orsborn G N, Walter C H, Knoll H A 1986 Studies on corneal staining with thin hydrogel contact lenses. J Br Contact Lens Assoc 9: 61–64

3

Corneal graft failure

D. G. C. Pendergrast   W. J. Armitage   C. A. Rogers   A. Vail
D. L. Easty

INTRODUCTION

Corneal grafting was first performed in 1906 and it has been considered a largely successful operation, but on scrutiny of the results in different types of disease this view is untenable. Corneal grafts are unique amongst transplants in that in addition to and in spite of technical, physiological, microbiological, immunological and pathological obstacles, the success of the transplant is finally determined by the visual result.

There are many reasons for graft failure and it is impossible to review each cause in this chapter. Those that present the greatest problems for the authors will be discussed. Since corneal graft rejection is one of the most common causes of failure, the immunological mechanisms and treatment will be discussed in detail.

FOLLOW-UP STUDIES

Success rates are based on transparency of the graft and final corrected visual acuity. Factors influencing these will be discussed under primary diagnosis, operative technique, early and late postoperative complications, allograft rejection, and quality of donor tissue. Case selection is important, and on occasions the prognosis is so poor that transplantation should not be considered.

Primary diagnosis

The results of grafting differ according to the primary diagnosis. Keratoconus, endothelial decompensation and inflammatory disease demonstrate widely differing results.

Keratoconus and other dystrophies

It is accepted that conditions where there is no corneal vascularization have a good prognosis, given good donor tissue and no operative complications. Keratoplasty for keratoconus has a success rate in the region of 95%, and acts as a bench mark for success rates in other conditions (Ehlers & Olsen 1983, Troutman & Lawless 1987).

Endothelial decompensation syndromes

Success rates in Fuchs' endothelial dystrophy are a further measure of basal complication rates, in that there is no corneal vascularization, although anterior segment inflammation is possible when severe corneal oedema occurs. However, Olsen et al (1984) report that visual acuity is less than 0.1 in 42% of cases, usually due to permanent graft oedema. It is likely that this graft failure is due to a lack of functional recipient endothelial cells, the donor cells sliding towards the peripheral host cornea, leading to eventual decompensation.

Success rates in pseudophakic or aphakic bullous keratopathy are unsatisfactory because there can be anterior segment inflammation preoperatively, and because of poor vision from cystoid macular oedema or age-related macular degeneration. Semi-flexible closed-loop anterior chamber lenses lead to poor visual results even when replaced with posterior chamber lenses at grafting (Insler et al 1989). Speaker et al (1988) recommend removal of closed loop implants and unstable lenses of any type, with well-fixated posterior chamber implants being left in situ. Most surgeons currently feel that the number of cases of bullous keratopathy are declining, probably due to the use of posterior chamber lenses and visco-elastic materials.

Inflammatory disease

Success rates in grafting for previous inflammatory disease such as herpes simplex keratitis are reduced in long-term follow-up studies. Ficker et al (1988), reviewing 65 patients with inflammatory disease after a mean follow-up period of 10.9 years, determined that the probability of survival is 45%, and that first grafts have a greater probability of success than second or further grafts.

Surgical technique

The technique aims at minimal manipulation of the donor tissue and attaining a watertight junction at the end of the procedure. It is not our intention to describe corneal grafting techniques in detail, but to highlight situations which lead to graft failure.

Globe fixation

In our experience significant improvements in results have come about from the use of the McNeill Goldmann ring, which consists of two scleral support rings and a blepharostat. This ring ensures good support of the whole recipient eye, which is drawn forward by the blepharostat, allowing the anterior chamber to be maintained easily without the use of excessive amounts of visco-elastic substances.

Trephine of donor and recipient

There are many modern trephines available but there is seemingly little to indicate that one has any particular advantage over another. When the donor tissue is cut from the endothelial surface, the size is smaller than when the procedure is carried out from the epithelial surface. A trephine 0.25–0.5 mm larger than the recipient bed is used to cut the donor tissue. This ensures a satisfactory and watertight interface, but disparity above 0.25 mm may increase astigmatism and induce postoperative myopia.

Suture management

Suturing must be accurate with good wound apposition to prevent loss of the anterior chamber or postoperative astigmatism. Many combinations are supported, including interrupted sutures, continuous suture plus interrupted, or two continuous sutures. Synechiae to the graft/host interface are frequently associated with allograft rejection, and their avoidance is critical. If regrafting is necessary the synechiae often return or even increase, again promoting rejection. Obviously iris should not be included in the interface, and to avoid this the anterior chamber should be reinflated regularly. At the end of the operation the interface must be watertight, and this can be checked by drying with a swab following re-formation of the anterior chamber. Leakage is easily seen, and if it is present extra sutures are required.

Astigmatism

Astigmatism is a common complication and may cause a poor visual result despite a clear graft. Predisposing factors are: severe preoperative astigmatism as in keratoconus, poor placement of donor button in relation to recipient aperture, incorrect placement of sutures or suture technique, postoperative suture erosion and use of an oversized rigid-loop anterior chamber implant. Scrupulous care in placement of the cardinal sutures is essential.

Operative keratometers vary in complexity but the simplest Placido's disc is satisfactory. However, despite good intraoperative keratometry, a significant amount of postoperative astigmatism may persist even following suture removal. Surgical correction is discussed below.

Early postoperative complications

The main early postoperative complications that may result in corneal graft failure are haemorrhage, infection, inflammation, wound leaks, epithelial defects and elevation of intraocular pressure.

Haemorrhage

Intraoperative bleeding may compromise the graft postoperatively. Significant haemorrhage may occur in severe anterior segment disorganization, or where there are extensive anterior synechiae following an earlier graft. Such haemorrhage is difficult to control and may spread into the vitreous in aphakia, where it may persist, particularly when visco-elastic substances have been used in large quantities. It can only be removed by vitrectomy. Bloodstaining of the graft is possible, and determines the need for operative intervention for its removal.

Infection

Bacterial infection is not uncommon and requires urgent investigation and treatment. There are a number of predisposing factors, such as contamination of the donor tissue (Panda et al 1988), intensive use of postoperative topical corticosteroid, eroding sutures causing stitch abscesses, persistent epithelial deficits, and recurrence of herpes simplex ulceration with secondary bacterial invasion. The recipient must be examined meticulously and treated for concurrent infective disease prior to surgery, a task that is occasionally taken too lightly where donor tissue is available and there is pressure to proceed.

Postoperative inflammation

Early re-establishment of the blood–aqueous barrier should reduce the possibility of systemic sensitization to MHC antigens and subsequent allograft rejection. The postoperative inflammatory response arises from the operative intervention, and occurs during the first 10–14 days. In many instances it is quite mild. In others, for example keratoconus with atopic conjunctivitis, the inflammation may be severe. Topical steroid is used initially. Where inflammation persists, systemic corticosteroid (say prednisolone 30 mg on alternate days) can be helpful.

Wound leaks

Meticulous attention to achieving a watertight interface between donor and recipient at the end of the surgery should avoid postoperative wound leaks. Where a leak does occur, it must be managed correctly, because anterior synechiae substantially increase the chance of allograft rejection. Where the anterior chamber is shallow and a leak is present extra sutures must be introduced within 24 hours.

Persistent epithelial deficit

This rare but important complication may lead to graft failure. It is seen in patients with dry eyes, mucous membrane disease such as pemphigoid and

Stevens–Johnson syndrome, in caustic burns and in anaesthetic corneas. Where there is significant pre-existing external eye disease the decision to perform surgery at all must be considered carefully because of the poor prognosis in such patients. If grafting is unavoidable, donor corneal epithelium should be retained, and fresh tissue from a young donor must be used. Immediately postoperatively, a high water content contact lens should be fitted to protect the epithelium until full recovery has taken place. Botulinum toxin-induced protective ptosis may also be considered (Kirkness et al 1988).

Pressure elevation

Postoperative glaucoma can be a cause of visual failure despite a clear graft. Visual loss may develop extremely rapidly so careful monitoring of pressure must rank as the most important measurement that is made in grafted patients.

Postoperative glaucoma can be related to the size disparity between donor and recipient trephines. Thus where donor is the same as recipient, there is narrowing of the angle, with increased incidence of glaucoma (Olson & Kaufman 1977, Bourne et al 1982). Where donor is larger than recipient, the evidence is conflicting. Zimmerman et al (1978) and Bourne et al (1982) found a lower pressure but other reports do not substantiate this (Foulks et al 1979, Perl et al 1981, Heidemann et al 1985). There is also evidence that large grafts, i.e. 8 mm or more in diameter, distort the angle and lead to higher postoperative intraocular pressure (Zimmerman et al 1978).

Late postoperative complications

The most important late postoperative complications are astigmatism and corneal graft rejection.

Surgical correction of astigmatism

This is indicated when astigmatism is unacceptable despite suture removal. For moderate astigmatism, say 5–10 dioptres, use relaxing incisions in the steepest meridian. Where there is in excess of 10 dioptres add compression sutures in the flatter meridian (MacCartney et al 1987). In excess of 6 dioptres decrease in astigmatism may be achieved (Mandel et al 1987), but with poor predictability in some cases (Lavery et al 1985), and more than one operation may be required (Price & Steele 1987). With refractory cases, wedge resection in the flattest meridian is carried out. Sutures are placed to close the two surfaces. This remains an effective and moderately predictable technique for managing high astigmatism following penetrating keratoplasty (Lugo et al 1987). Potential refinements in technique are promised from computerized imaging of the corneal surface, producing a dioptric colour-coded contour map of corneal surface powers (Dingeldein & Klyce 1988).

The surgeon must be absolutely certain that the incision and sutures are appropriately placed; errors of 90° are easily made. To prevent this a diagram should be drawn and consulted during surgery.

IMMUNOLOGICAL GRAFT REJECTION

Transplant immunology

Transplants between genetically different individuals are rejected largely because of differences between donor and recipient in the structure of polymorphic glycoproteins on the surface of their cells. The genetic loci controlling these histocompatibility antigens is referred to as the major histocompatibility complex (MHC). Other minor histocompatibility loci code for antigens evoking a weaker rejection response. The human MHC is the human leucocyte antigen (HLA) complex, a group of genetic loci on the short arm of chromosome 6.

The HLA system

The HLA loci and molecules are divided into two classes on the basis of tissue distribution, structure and function. Class I molecules are expressed by virtually all nucleated cells. They are composed of a heavy α-chain glycoprotein, variable between individuals and encoded in the HLA complex; this is bound to a β_2-microglobulin, an invariant light-chain polypeptide encoded on chromosome 15 (Fig. 3.1). There are three Class I loci: HLA-A, HLA-B and HLA-C. HLA-C molecules are elements of the complement cascade and will not be discussed further.

Class II molecules have a tissue distribution limited to cells involved directly with the immune response. They are normally expressed by B lymphocytes and by antigen-presenting cells (APC) such as dendritic cells and tissue macrophages. They are composed of two glycoproteins: an α-chain and a β-chain, both encoded within the HLA complex (Fig. 3.1). There are three class II loci: HLA-DR, HLA-DQ and HLA-DP. The extent of Class II expression on cells is not fixed but can be up- and down-regulated.

These genes are very polymorphic; more than 125 HLA specificities are presently recognized. Most persons are heterozygous and express six different molecules of each class.

The importance of the HLA system has become apparent with the realization that a necessary step in sensitization to foreign antigen is the activation of helper T cells, and that this activation is not induced by antigen alone but requires this antigen to be presented on the surface of an APC in association with a Class II HLA molecule. This is described as MHC restriction.

HLA molecules bind antigenic peptides. Two-dimensional crystallographic studies of HLA-A2 have shown a deep groove between the α_1 and the α_2 domains on the top surface of the molecule, containing electron-dense

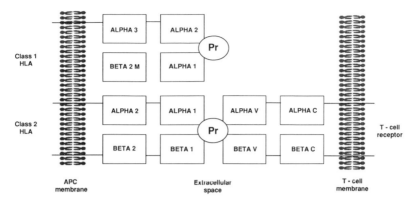

Fig. 3.1 HLA molecules and the T cell receptor (diagrammatic). Alpha 1,2,3: polypeptide domains within the α-glycoprotein chain of the HLA molecule. Beta 2 M: β_2-microglobulin of the Class I HLA molecule. Alpha V, beta V: variable regions of the T cell receptor. Alpha C, beta C: constant regions of the T cell receptor. P: antigenic peptide bound to the HLA molecule.

material postulated to be bound peptide (Bjorkman et al 1987). A majority of the amino acid substitutions between different alleles of a given HLA type that alter T cell recognition face into this binding site.

T cell activation

HLA molecules and antigen on the surface of the APC interact with T cell receptors (Fig. 3.1). These cell surface polypeptides contain constant and variable regions, and it is the latter that are involved in specific antigen recognition. The most highly polymorphic areas of the variable regions contact bound peptide in the antigen-binding groove, while other parts of the receptor contact the HLA molecule itself (Davis & Bjorkman 1988).

Other cell surface molecules are also involved and differ according to the type of T cell involved. Monoclonal antibodies to these molecules can be used to identify T cell subsets. CD4 is found on the surface of helper/inducer T cells and these cells bind preferentially to Class II HLA molecules. CD8 is found on the surface of cytotoxic/suppressor T cells and these cells bind preferentially to Class I HLA molecules.

The interaction between the T cell receptor and specific antigen results in the formation of at least two intracellular second messengers, inositol triphosphate and diacylglycerol. These then induce a rise in cytoplasmic free calcium, and activation of protein kinase C and tyrosine kinase (Weiss & Imboden 1987). Subsequent genetic regulatory events resulting from these changes lead to T cell activation (Krensky et al 1990). Interleukin-2 production is induced and also the expression of interleukin-2 receptors. This is essential for T cell proliferation and affects both the activated cell and other cells. Interleukin-3 is produced and stimulates the proliferation of stem cells.

Interleukins 4, 5 and 6, B cell growth and differentiation factors are produced. Gamma interferon is produced and increases the expression of Class I and Class II HLA antigens as well as enhancing the activity of antigen-non-specific effector cells such as macrophages and natural killer cells (Irschick et al 1989).

The immune response in the cornea

Corneal HLA expression

Human cornea expresses HLA Class I antigens on epithelial, stromal and corneal endothelial cells and on the endothelial cells lining limbal blood vessels (Abu El-Asrar et al 1989). In the epithelium there is a gradient of expression that increases towards the periphery. HLA Class II expression is restricted to dendritic cells in the epithelium and corneal stroma. The epithelial dendritic cells are more frequent towards the periphery, the stromal cells are more evenly distributed (Treseler et al 1984).

The epithelial dendritic cells are a distinct population of wandering cells of mesenchymal origin that are equivalent to the Langerhans cells of the epidermis and, sharing many of their characteristics, are referred to as corneal Langerhans cells (Gillette et al 1982). The dendritic cells of the corneal stroma are similar. These cells are recognized as playing a central role as antigen presenting cells in corneal graft rejection (Williams & Coster 1989).

Class II expression has been induced on human corneal epithelial, stromal and endothelial cells in vitro by the lymphokine gamma interferon (Dreizen et al 1988, Abu El-Asrar et al 1989) and in vivo in rabbits by experimental uveitis (Donnelly et al 1985).

Graft destruction

Following activation of CD4 + helper T cells the events described above lead to the production and activation of CD8 + cytotoxic T cells. These cells attack specifically donor cells bearing Class I HLA and the sensitizing antigen. There may also be a population of CD4 + cytotoxic T cells directed against Class II bearing cells. In addition to these antigen-specific attacks there are also other leucocytes found in rejecting grafts and natural killer cells may cause some graft damage non-specifically during episodes of ocular inflammation.

The role of humoral immunity in corneal graft rejection is uncertain. Donor-specific cytotoxic antibody has been shown to be produced following experimental heterotopic corneal graft rejection (Treseler & Sanfilippo 1985). Also the absence of preformed antibodies against donor antigens is associated with a reduced rate of graft rejection (Stark et al 1978). Direct evidence of antibody-mediated graft damage in humans is lacking.

Direct antigen presentation

In graft rejection the sensitization of the host is mainly dependent on the presence of donor APC carrying foreign Class II HLA molecules and capable of secreting interleukin-1 and thus activating host resting T cells. The nature of the recognition of foreign HLA by T cells is not clearly understood but it is thought to be a cross-reaction occurring because the structure of non-self HLA molecule resembles that of self-HLA plus antigen. Strategies that affect the numbers of APC in a graft have been shown to influence graft survival in other organ systems (Lafferty 1980).

Indirect antigen presentation

Host antigen-presenting cells can also take up and present donor MHC antigens (Sherwood et al 1986). Graft damage by effector cells would, however, not be expected since the cytotoxic T cells should not recognize the sensitizing antigens except in the context of self MHC molecules. A relationship has nevertheless been shown between the incidence of graft failure and the number of dendritic cells in the recipient corneal tissue (Williams & Coster 1989), and a number of workers (Williams et al 1987b, Peeler & Niederkorn 1987) have suggested that with partial HLA compatibility indirect processing of donor antigen by host dendritic cells could result in specific as well as non-specific damage to graft cells. Attempts at dendritic cell depletion should thus be directed at the recipient as well as the donor.

In the case of total MHC identity between donor and host both donor and host APC may present minor histocompatibility antigens to host T cells (Loveland & Simpson 1987). Recent work in our own laboratory confirms that isotopic corneal transplants between rats identical at Class I and II loci but differing at minor histocompatibility loci nevertheless reject, although with a reduced tempo (Nicholls Bradley & Easty 1990).

Risk factors for graft rejection

In theory, graft rejection may be prevented by reducing the antigenicity of the donor material, by minimizing the antigenic differences between donor and recipient, and by interfering with the sensitization and activation of the host immune response. Certain donor and host factors, some of which may be manipulated, have been identified as influencing the risk of graft rejection.

Donor factors

Organ culture. In other organ systems prolonged storage in tissue culture medium reduces the numbers of APC and reduces the incidence of graft rejection. Storage in organ culture for greater than one week causes the disappearance of Langerhans cells from corneal epithelium (Holland et al 1987) associated with partial sloughing of the epithelium. Patients receiving an organ-cultured cornea have a significantly better graft survival than those receiving a moist pot or McCarey–Kaufman stored cornea (Volker-Dieben et al 1987). This may of course relate to other factors such as endothelial cell survival.

Ultraviolet light. In experimental animals a reduction in the incidence of corneal allograft rejection has been produced by exposure of the donor tissue to ultraviolet light. This appears to be due to the reduction in numbers or activity of Langerhans cells that results (Guymer & Mandel 1989). These findings have not yet been applied to human grafting.

Graft size. The effect of graft size on the incidence of rejection is controversial. A small button will contain fewer Class II expressing Langerhans cells and thus less stimulus to rejection. In addition the graft–host junction will be further from the recipient limbus with its concentration of host APCs and blood vessels. Two large studies (Volker-Dieben et al 1987, Boisjoly et al 1989) confirm that larger grafts do less well than smaller grafts.

Removal of donor epithelium. Donor epithelium contains greater than 90% of the nucleated cells of the cornea and its removal has been suggested as a way to reduce the antigenic load of the donor material. Although some Langerhans cells would be removed with the epithelium, Class II positive APC have also been found in the stroma of normal human corneas (Treseler et al 1984, Abu El-Asrar et al 1989). In comparison to Class I positive, Class II negative epidermal cells, Langerhans cells have an extraordinary capacity to sensitize a recipient to alloantigens (McKinney & Streilein 1989). Tuberville et al (1983) in a mixed retrospective and prospective clinical study supported removal of epithelium. A more recent prospective randomized clinical trial (Stulting et al 1987) was unable to demonstrate any reduction in graft rejection following removal of donor epithelium. At least on theoretical grounds removal of epithelium is probably not justified.

Host factors

Vascularization. There is a significant association between severe vascularization of the recipient cornea and irreversible graft rejection (Batchelor et al 1976, Volker-Dieben et al 1987, Boisjoly et al 1989). Increased numbers of Langerhans cells are present in vascularized corneas (Williams et al 1985a) and host sensitization will occur rapidly.

Inflammation. The number of Langerhans cells in the cornea is also increased by inflammation and previous graft rejection (Gillette et al 1982, Williams et al 1985a). Class II antigen expression on epithelial and endothelial cells may be induced by inflammatory processes within the eye and this may explain why inflammatory events such as infection may trigger graft rejection.

Previous sensitization. Pre-graft sensitization to the HLA antigens of the donor may be the cause of the increased risk of rejection following previous grafting (Batchelor et al 1976, Sanfilippo et al 1986, Volker-Dieben et al 1987,

Boisjoly et al 1989) but given the polymorphism of the HLA system the chance of sensitization to one of the antigens of the new donor is low. Possibly it is the corneal vascularization resulting from rejection that actually leads to this risk. Previous pregnancy or blood transfusion does not appear to have a significant influence on graft rejection rate (Volker-Dieben et al 1987, Boisjoly et al 1989).

Factors of both donor and recipient

HLA matching. Several studies have supported the value of Class I HLA matching in high-risk cases, generally defined as previous graft rejection or a severely vascularized cornea (Batchelor et al 1976, Sanfilippo et al 1986, Volker-Dieben et al 1987). In recipients with no vascularization of their corneas HLA matching appears to have no effect on prognosis.

The effect of HLA Class II matching has not been as extensively studied (Boisjoly et al 1986, Volker-Dieben et al 1987) but increasing knowledge of the role of the APC in corneal graft rejection suggests that it will be found to be of importance.

The Corneal Transplant Service Follow-up Study in the UK gathers and analyses data from many centres, assessing survival of all corneal transplants at three months, 12 months, and then yearly. One of the main objectives is to evaluate prospectively HLA matching. To date the accrual is 2302 grafts, with three-month follow-up data in 812. Table 3.1 shows the breakdown by primary diagnosis. The main influences on final visual acuity are shown in Fig. 3.2, where the results in keratoconus are used as the baseline for determination of the relative rates in other conditions (Easty et al 1990).

Similar studies are being carried out in selected centres in the USA (Stark et al 1989), Australia (Williams et al 1987a) and Amsterdam (Volker-Dieben et al 1987).

ABO matching. Most studies suggest that ABO incompatibility does not influence graft prognosis (Allansmith et al 1975, Batchelor et al 1976) despite the demonstration of blood group antigens on both epithelium and endothelium of human cornea (Salisbury & Gebhardt 1981, Treseler et al 1986).

Table 3.1 Primary diagnosis in grafts included in the Corneal Transplant Follow-up Study

Primary diagnosis	Incidence (%)	Mean age (SD)
Inflammation	23	59 (17.2)
Secondary endothelial failure	23	69 (15.5)
Keratoconus	20	36 (11.9)
Primary endothelial failure	13	69 (15.6)
Stromal dystrophy	5	57 (19.8)
Trauma	4	42 (20.2)
Other	11	56 (22.6)

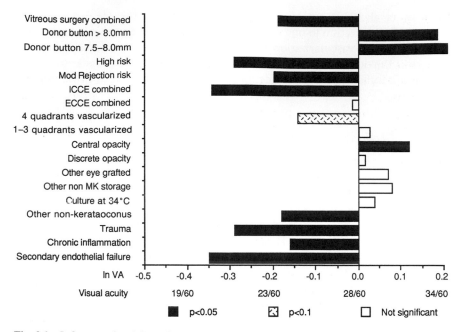

Fig. 3.2 Influence of recipient, donor and surgical factors on visual acuity at three months. Visual acuity is expressed on a logarithmic scale and compared with a baseline (keratoconus, no corneal vascularization, MK storage at 4°C, donor <7.5 mm and no cataract extraction or vitreous surgery performed). Significantly worse acuity is found with grafting for other diseases shown here in comparison to keratoconus. Cataract extraction or vitreous surgery combined with the graft also significantly affects results. The result for a given patient can be predicted by adding their individual risk scores to baseline. For example a patient with secondary endothelial failure (– 0.35), receiving a cultured cornea (+ 0.04), with 1–3 quadrants of vascularization (+ 0.03), and a donor size of 7.5–8.0 mm (+ 0.21); total deviation from baseline is – 0.09, corresponding to an acuity of between 23/60 and 28/60.

Race. This factor has not been extensively studied. The incidence of different HLA serotypes varies between races; however, one retrospective study (Musch et al 1988) on 998 grafts found no significant difference in risk of endothelial rejection between race-matched and race-mismatched recipients, both for low- and high-risk cases.

Pharmacological immunosuppression

Pharmacological immunosuppression may prevent recipient sensitization or if it has occurred may reduce T cell activation and division.

Corticosteroids

Corticosteroids inhibit early gene activation events in T cells (Krensky et al 1990) by acting on short segments of DNA called response elements. The result is inhibition of T cell proliferation. In addition they inhibit the angiogenic process. Depletion of corneal Langerhans cells by either topical or systemic corticosteroid treatment has been demonstrated in an animal model (Gillette et al 1982).

Preoperative topical corticosteroids, if not contraindicated, should be used for several days in eyes at risk of graft rejection. Postoperatively topical corticosteroids are widely used and in high-risk cases are mandatory and should be continued for several months. Systemic corticosteroids may also be used in high-risk cases in doses of 20–30 mg prednisolone per day. Because of the complications of long-term use, it is desirable to reduce the dose of systemic corticosteroids, if possible, and combination therapy with another immunosuppressive agent such as azathioprine or cyclosporin A may allow more effective therapy with fewer side-effects.

Once rejection has begun, rapid aggressive treatment may minimize immunological damage to the graft and induce rapid resolution. Patients must be taught the symptoms and signs of possible graft rejection and are strongly advised to present quickly if they develop. If the graft rejection is in its early stages, topical steroid therapy may halt the destructive process. The patient should be admitted to hospital and given potent steroid drops at least hourly. Subconjunctival and systemic steroids may also be used in more severe graft rejection. After two to three weeks the systemic medication may be reduced and topical therapy continued.

Azathioprine

Azathioprine acts non-specifically by impeding proliferation of rapidly dividing cells, including lymphoid cells. Its use has been advocated (Barraquer 1985, Coster 1989) in high-risk keratoplasty. It is useful in combination with systemic corticosteroids to allow a reduction in steroid dose. An effective maintenance dose is 1–2 mg/kg per day. Careful monitoring of the haematopoietic system, liver and renal function is necessary, with reduction or cessation of treatment if toxicity develops.

Cyclosporin A (CSA)

CSA is a potent immunosuppressive agent with a high degree of specificity for T lymphocytes and has been widely used systemically to induce tolerance to allografts. The mechanism is not fully known and may involve several factors. CSA acts on helper T lymphocytes to inhibit the release of interleukin-1, interleukin-2 and gamma interferon, inhibiting activation of the host immune response. CSA selectively spares suppressor T cells (Kupiec-Weglinski et al 1984), which renders the host tolerant towards allografted tissues. Miller et al (1988) have successfully used CSA to prevent rejection in high risk corneal allografts in humans, and on examining numbers of T cell precursors in peripheral blood (Irschick et al 1989) conclude that tolerance is not caused by any reduction in the clone size of donor-specific cytotoxic T cells.

Systemic use. Animal models support the use of CSA in the prevention of corneal graft rejection (Bell et al 1982). Hill (1989) describes its clinical use in high-risk keratoplasty and concludes that the combination of CSA, systemic and topical steroids significantly increased graft survival compared to steroids alone. CSA dose was adjusted to maintain a therapeutic level of 250–400 μg/l of whole blood with the usual dose being 4.0–4.5 mg/kg of body weight per day. There were no permanent side-effects related to the use of CSA.

Despite its potential for nephrotoxicity, if used at a dose of 5.0 mg/kg and with careful monitoring of renal function and blood levels, CSA appears to have a definite use in the prevention of graft rejection in recipients with vascularized corneas. The dangers of systemic use must, however, be considered and it is perhaps best reserved for cases where a successful outcome is imperative such as repeat grafting in an only eye.

Topical use. Topical CSA has been shown in animal models to delay corneal graft rejection but grafts reject when it is stopped (Kana et al 1982, Hunter et al 1982). Combined topical CSA and steroid is no more effective than steroid alone in preventing rejection of rat corneal allografts (Williams et al 1987c) and topical CSA alone is less effective than topical steroid (Williams et al 1985b). Because of the insolubility of CSA in water a commercial preparation of CSA in drop form is not available. Recently an ointment has been manufactured; multicentred trials of use in corneal graft rejection are planned. CSA is unlikely to add much to current topical therapy for the prevention of corneal graft rejection.

IMPROVING THE QUALITY OF DONOR MATERIAL

The development of centralized eye banks is a significant recent advance and has resulted in improvements in corneal donor tissue quality and supply. The Bristol-based Corneal Transplant Service Eye Bank is described as an example of the banks now operating in several countries.

The Corneal Transplant Service Eye Bank (CTSEB)

In September 1983 a National Corneal Transplant Service (CTS) was inaugurated, with a grant from the Iris Fund for the Prevention of Blindness, at the Bristol-based UK Transplant Service (UKTS). The aims were to broaden the field of potential donors by increasing awareness, to coordinate the use of available donor corneas, to obviate waste of surplus corneal tissue and, where applicable, to reduce the incidence of rejection by the provision of tissue-matched corneas. UKTS provides McCarey–Kaufman medium, sterile eye containers, disposable eye stands and transportation boxes to hospitals that require them. Redistribution of corneas via a 24-hour on-call matching and transport service avoids waste. A national corneal waiting list is maintained and statistical analysis for administrative and scientific purposes is carried out.

The waiting list for corneas rose faster than for any other organ during 1985, and now appears to be reaching a steady state at approximately 600 patients (Fig. 3.3). In excess of 100 centres have now registered patients with UKTS and over 150 have either received or contributed tissue to the Corneal Transplant Service. The number of corneal transplants which have been reported to UKTS has risen between 1984 and 1990 from approximately 400 to well in excess of 1500 (Fig. 3.4).

In collaboration with the Department of Ophthalmology at the University of Bristol, the CTSEB was established at UKTS in 1986. Clinical trials of various corneal storage techniques are conducted through the bank, which supplies corneas to an increasing number of operating surgeons within the UK. In 1989 1500 organ culture stored corneas were supplied to over 100 hospitals within the British Isles (Fig. 3.5).

Methods of corneal storage

Many workers have contributed to the development of the techniques of corneal storage that make this service possible. The advantages and disavantages of these various techniques are described below.

Short-term storage

Donor eyes may be stored in a moist chamber at 4°C for up to 48 hours (Filatov 1937). However, even within this interval signs of endothelial stress

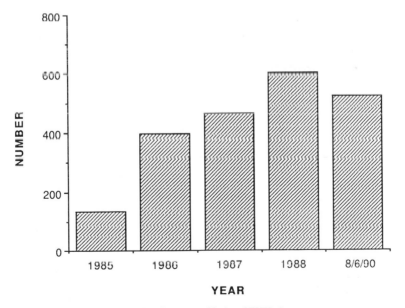

Fig. 3.3 Corneal transplant waiting list, as notified to UKTS, by year.

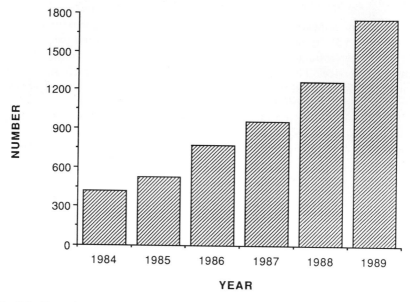

Fig. 3.4 Corneal transplants notified to UKTS, by year.

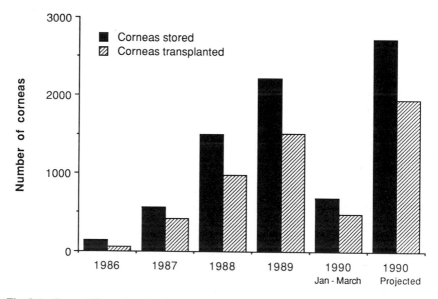

Fig. 3.5 Corneal Transplant Service Eye Bank activity, by year. 1990 figures are projected from figures for the first quarter.

occur, with some collapse of the cell and the appearance of granular changes on the cell membrane.

McCarey–Kaufman medium

Extended corneal storage at 4°C has come about as a result of the availability of standard tissue culture media, which developed from the work of Eagle in 1955. A well-tried and highly successful technique for short-term storage involves the use of tissue culture medium containing 5% dextran (McCarey & Kaufman 1974), which allows preservation for up to four days (Van Horn & Schultz 1977), permitting greater flexibility in scheduling surgery. The use of hyperosmotic dextran in the M–K solution maintains the disc in a deturgescent state which facilitates surgery. It is necessary to remove the corneo-scleral disc from the donor eye soon after death, using sterile technique, either in a laminar flow cabinet in a properly designed eye bank, or within the operating theatre. Scanning electron microscopy shows that the technique is dependable and that it is probably superior to the use of moist chambers.

A useful modification of this medium occurred when it was found that inclusion of chondroitin sulphate (such as in K-sol) extended the storage time. The first reports suggested that up to 14 days of storage was safe (Kaufman et al 1985). However, postoperative loss of endothelial cells increases with increasing storage time in both K Sol and M–K medium, and Bourne (1986) suggested that corneas should be stored for no more than ten days in K-Sol. It should be noted that the average donor age in Bourne's study was only 35 years and the corneas were retrieved within six hours of death of the donors; older donor age and a longer interval between donor death and corneal removal are likely to limit further the permissible storage period.

Organ culture

The storage of corneas in tissue culture medium at 34–37°C allows up to 30 days storage compared with the two to four days permitted at 4°C. This method has proved to be a significant advance in corneal storage (Doughman et al 1976, Pels & Schuchard 1983). Apart from any difference in the tissue itself, HIV-infected donors can be excluded and storage for several weeks simplifies the logistics of finding suitably matched donor–recipient pairs. In addition, with fresh tissue viable pre-mortem lymphocytes are often not available for tissue typing. With the increased time before tissue use, tissue culture of donor retinal pigment epithelial cells can be used to obtain cells suitable for HLA typing (Baumgartner et al 1989).

The methodology must be followed with scrupulous care (Easty et al 1986, Armitage & Moss 1990). After enucleation the globe is cleaned, and the corneo-scleral disc removed and incubated in 60 ml tissue culture medium at 34°C. After seven days 1 ml of medium is removed for microbiological screening for fungi and bacteria. If the culture is not contaminated, it is left until two days before elective surgery is planned, and then prepared for use. The endothelium is stained with trypan blue and examined by light microscopy. If the count is low due to excessive cell death or loss the cornea is discarded. Corneas become oedematous during organ culture. Following endothelial microscopy, they are placed in medium containing 5% dextran, which thins them prior to transplantation (Pels & Schuchard 1983). The cornea must now be kept at room temperature or above: if organ-cultured corneas are subsequently placed at 4°C, even for only a few hours, postoperative loss of endothelial cells is exacerbated (Bourne et al 1985).

Ten donor corneas stored in Bristol in organ culture have been examined by specular microscopy at two, six and 12 months following transplantation (Fig. 3.6). The average loss of endothelial cells between two and 12 months was 14.4% This loss rate is very similar to that reported by Bourne (1983) for a much larger series of grafts using corneas stored at 4°C in M–K medium. From a clinical point of view, the stroma takes longer to deturgesce, with more folds in Descemet's membrane compared to fresh tissue. However, so far experience suggests that the final visual result does not differ from that obtained with fresh tissue.

KEY POINTS TO CLINICAL PRACTICE

1.   The results of grafting differ according to the primary diagnosis. In some cases the prognosis is so poor that transplant should not be considered.

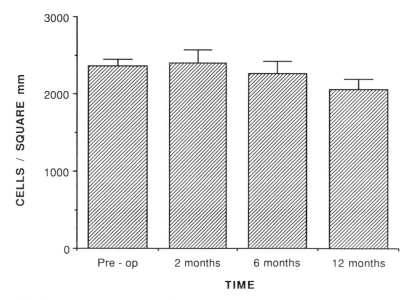

Fig. 3.6   Pre- and postoperative endothelial cell densities of organ cultured corneas (mean ± SEM, $n = 10$) (Armitage & Moss 1990).

2. Preoperative identification and treatment of any concurrent infective or inflammatory disease is essential.

3. The aims of surgical technique are minimal manipulation of the donor tissue and careful suture placement to avoid wound leak or astigmatism.

4. Visual results are too often poor despite a clear graft. Glaucoma and astigmatism must be looked for and treated aggressively.

5. Organ culture storage of donor corneas is an important advance and allows improved donor tissue quality and supply.

6. Increasing knowledge of the mechanisms of allograft rejection suggests that HLA matching should be of benefit. This is not yet conclusively proven in clinical trials.

7. Pharmacological immune suppression is important in all cases. Intensity and duration should be influenced by preoperative, operative and postoperative factors known to increase the risk of immunological graft rejection. Corticosteroids are first-line agents. Therapeutic effect may be increased and side-effects decreased by the addition of other immunosuppressives.

8. Early and aggressive treatment of rejection episodes will reduce the tissue damage and improve graft survival. Patient education is important.

ACKNOWLEDGEMENTS

Professor B. A. Bradley (Director UKTS) was instrumental in the initiation of the Corneal Transplant Service Follow-up Study. Dr S. M. Moss (Research Fellow, Department of Ophthalmology, University of Bristol) and Dr S. M. Gore (Biostatistician, MRC Biostatistics Unit, Cambridge) are acknowledged for data collection and interpretation. Endothelial cell counts in Fig. 3.1 were carried out by Mr R. M. Redmond.

Financial support for this work was provided by the Smith and Nephew Foundation, the National Eye Research Centre, the Iris Fund for the Prevention of Blindness and the Small Grants Committee of the DHSS.

REFERENCES

Abu El-Asrar A M, Van Den Oord J J, Billiau A et al 1989 Recombinant interferon-gamma induces HLA-DR expression on human corneal epithelial and endothelial cells in vitro: a preliminary report. Br J Ophthalmol 73: 587–590
Allansmith M R, Drew D W, Kajiyama G et al 1975 ABO blood groups and corneal transplantation. Am J Ophthalmol 79: 493–501
Armitage W J, Moss S J 1990 Storage of corneas for transplantation. In: Easty D L (ed) Current ophthalmic surgery. Baillière-Tindall, London
Barraquer J 1985 Immunosuppressive agents in penetrating keratoplasty. Am J Ophthalmol 100: 61–64
Batchelor J R, Casey T A, Gibbs D C et al 1976 HLA matching and corneal grafting. Lancet i: 551–554

Baumgartner I, Mayr W R, Grabner G 1989 Corneal grafting-strategy for optimal results. Tissue Antigens 34: 5–8

Bell T A, Easty D L, McCullagh K G 1982 A placebo controlled blind trial of cyclosporin-A in prevention of corneal graft rejection in rabbits. Br J Ophthalmol 66: 303–308

Bjorkman P J, Saper M A, Samraoui B et al 1987 The foreign antigen binding site and T cell recognition regions of class I histocompatibility antigens. Nature 329: 512–518

Boisjoly H M, Roy R, Dube I et al 1986 HLA A, B and DR matching in corneal transplantation. Ophthalmology 93: 1290–1297

Boisjoly H M, Bernard P, Dube I et al 1989 Effect of factors unrelated to tissue matching on corneal transplant endothelial rejection. Am J Ophthalmol 107: 647–654

Bourne W M 1983 Chronic endothelial cell loss in transplanted corneas. Cornea 2: 289–294

Bourne W M 1986 Endothelial cell survival on transplanted human corneas preserved at 4°C in 2.5% chondroitin sulfate for 1 to 13 days. Am J Ophthalmol 102: 382–386

Bourne W, Davison J, O'Fallon W 1982 The effects of oversize donor buttons on postoperative intraocular pressure and corneal curvature in aphakic penetrating keratoplasty. Ophthalmology 89: 242–246

Bourne W M, Doughman D J, Lindstrom R L 1985 Decreased endothelial cell survival after transplantation of corneas preserved by three modifications of the organ culture technique. Ophthalmology 92: 1538–1541

Coster D J 1989 Mechanisms of corneal graft failure: the erosion of corneal privilege. Eye 2: 251–262

Davis M M, Bjorkman P J 1988 T-cell receptor genes and T-cell recognition. Nature 334: 395–402

Dingeldein S A, Klyce S D 1988 Imaging of the cornea. Cornea 7: 170–182

Donnelly J J, Li W, Rockey J H, Prendergast R A 1985 Induction of class II (Ia) alloantigen expression on corneal endothelium in vivo and in vitro. Invest Ophthalmol Vis Sci 26: 575–580

Doughman D J, Harris J E, Schmitt M K 1976 Penetrating keratoplasty using 37°C organ cultured corneas. Trans Am Acad Ophthalmol Otolaryngol 81: 778–793

Dreizen N G, Whitsett C F, Stulting R D 1988 Modulation of HLA antigen expression on corneal epithelial and stromal cells. Invest Ophthalmol Vis Sci 29: 933–939

Easty D L, Carter C A, Lewkowicz-Moss S J 1986 Corneal cell culture and organ storage. Trans Ophthalmol Soc UK 105: 385–396

Easty D L, Rogers C A, Gore S M et al 1990 Corneal transplant follow-up study (CTFS). Invest Ophthalmol Vis Sci 31: 270

Ehlers N, Olsen T 1983 Long term results of corneal grafting in keratoconus. Acta Ophthalmol 61: 918–926

Ficker L A, Kirkness C M, Rice N S et al 1988 Longterm prognosis for corneal grafting in herpes simplex keratitis. Eye 2: 400–408

Filatov V P 1937 Transplantation of the cornea from preserved cadaver: eyes. Lancet i: 1395–1397

Foulks G N, Perry H D, Dohlman C H 1979 Oversize corneal donor grafts in penetrating keratoplasty. Ophthalmology 86: 490–494

Gillette T E, Chandler J W, Greiner J V 1982 Langerhans' cells of the ocular surface. Ophthalmology 89: 700–710

Guymer R H, Mandel T E 1989 UV-B irradiation of donor skin and cornea prior to allotransplantation in mice. Transplant Proc 21: 3771–3772

Heidemann D G, Sugar A, Meyer R F et al 1985 Oversized donor grafts in penetrating keratoplasty: a randomized trial. Arch Ophthalmol 103: 1807–1811

Hill J C 1989 The use of cyclosporine in high-risk keratoplasty. Am J Ophthalmol 107: 506–510

Holland E J, DeRuyter D N, Doughman D J 1987 Langerhans' cells in organ cultured corneas. Arch Ophthalmol 105: 542–545

Hunter P A, Garner A, Wilhelmus K R et al 1982 Corneal graft rejection: a new rabbit model and cyclosporin-A. Br J Ophthalmol 66: 292–302

Insler M S, Kook M S, Kaufman H E 1989 Penetrating keratoplasty for pseudophakic bullous keratopathy associated with semiflexible, closed-loop anterior chamber intraocular lenses. Am J Ophthalmol 107: 252–256

Irschick E, Miller K, Berger M et al 1989 Studies of the mechanism of tolerance induced by short-term immunosuppression with cyclosporine in high-risk corneal allograft recipients. Transplantation 48: 986–990

Kana J S, Hoffmann F, Buchen R et al 1982 Rabbit corneal allograft survival following topical administration of cyclosporin A. Invest Ophthalmol Vis Sci 22: 686–690

Kaufman H E, Varnell E D, Kaufman S et al 1985 K-Sol corneal preservation. Am J Ophthalmol 100: 299–304

Kirkness C M, Adams G G W, Dilly P N et al 1988 Botulinum toxin A induced protective ptosis in corneal disease. Ophthalmology 95: 473–480

Koenig S B, McDermott M L, Hyndiuk R A 1989 Penetrating keratoplasty and intraocular lens exchange for pseudophakic bullous keratopathy associated with a closed-loop anterior chamber intraocular lens. Am J Ophthalmol 108: 43–48

Krensky A M, Weiss A, Crabtree G et al 1990 T-lymphocyte–antigen interaction in transplant rejection. N Engl J Med 322: 510–517

Kupiec-Weglinski J W, Filho M A, Strom T B et al 1984 Sparing of suppressor cells: a critical action of cyclosporine. Transplantation 38: 97–100

Lafferty K J 1980 Immunogenicity of foreign tissues. Transplantation 29: 179–182

Lavery G W, Lindstrom R L, Hofer L A et al 1985 The surgical management of corneal astigmatism after penetrating keratoplasty. Ophthalmic Surg 16: 165–169

Limberg M B, Dingeldein S A, Green M T et al 1989 Corneal compression sutures for the reduction of astigmatism after penetrating keratoplasty. Am J Ophthalmol 108: 36–42

Loveland B, Simpson E 1986 The non-MHC transplantation antigens: neither weak nor minor. Immunol Today 7: 223–229

Lugo M, Donnenfeld E D, Arenstsen J J 1987 Corneal wedge resection for high astigmatism following penetrating keratoplasty. Ophthalmic Surg 18: 650–653

MacCartney D L, Whitney C E, Stark W J et al 1987 Refractive keratoplasty for disabling astigmatism after penetrating keratoplasty. Arch Ophthalmol 105: 954–957

Mandel M R, Shapiro M B, Krachmer J H 1987 Relaxing incisions with augmentation sutures for the correction of postkeratoplasty astigmatism. Am J Ophthalmol 103: 441–447

McCarey B E, Kaufman H E 1974 Improved corneal storage. Invest Ophthalmol Vis Sci 13: 165–173

McKinney E C, Streilein J W 1989 On the extraordinary capacity of allogeneic epidermal Langerhans cells to prime cytotoxic T cells in vivo. J Immunol 143: 1560–1564

Miller K, Huber C, Niederwieser D et al 1988 Successful engraftment of high-risk corneal allografts with short-term immunosuppression with cyclosporine. Transplantation 45: 651–653

Musch D C, Meyer R F, Sugar A et al 1988 A study of race matching between donor and recipient in corneal transplantation. Am J Ophthalmol 105: 646–650

Nicholls S, Bradley B A, Easty D L 1991 The role of MHC and non MHC antigens on corneal graft rejection. Invest ophthalmol vis Sci (in press)

Olsen T, Ehlers N, Favini E 1984 Long term results of corneal grafting in Fuchs' endothelial dystrophy. Acta Ophthalmol 63: 445–452

Olson R J, Kaufman H E 1977 A mathematical description of causative factors and prevention of elevated intraocular pressure after keratoplasty. Invest Ophthalmol Vis Sci 16: 1085–1092

Panda A, Angra S K, Venkateshwarlu K et al 1988 Microbial contamination of donor eyes. Jpn J Ophthalmol 32: 264–267

Peeler J S, Niederkorn J Y 1987 Effect of Langerhans' cells on cytotoxic T lymphocyte responses to major and minor alloantigens expressed on heterotopic corneal allografts. Transplant Proc 19: 316–319

Pels E, Schuchard Y 1983 Organ-culture preservation of human corneas. Doc Ophthalmol 56: 147–153

Perl T, Charlton K, Binder P 1981 Disparate diameter grafting: astigmatism, intraocular pressure, and visual acuity. Ophthalmology 88: 774–781

Price N C, Steele A D McG 1987 The correction of post-keratoplasty astigmatism. Eye 1: 562–566

Salisbury J D, Gebhardt M 1981 Blood group antigens on human corneal cells demonstrated by immunoperoxidase staining. Am J Ophthalmol 91: 46–50

Sanfilippo F, MacQueen J M, Vaughn W K et al 1986 Reduced graft rejection with good HLA-A and B matching in high-risk corneal transplantation. N Engl J Med 315: 29–35

Sherwood R A, Brent L, Rayfield L S 1986 Presentation of alloantigens by host cells. Eur J Immunol 16: 569–574

Speaker M G, Lugo M, Laibson P R et al 1988 Penetrating keratoplasty for pseudophakic bullous keratopathy. Management of the intra-ocular lens. Ophthalmology 95: 1260–1268

Stark W J, Taylor H R, Bias W B et al 1978 Histocompatibility (HLA) antigens and keratoplasty. Am J Ophthalmol 86: 595–604

Stark W J, Stulting R D, Meyer R F et al 1989 Sharing tissue typing information from the collaborative corneal transplantation studies. Arch Ophthalmol 107: 633

Stulting R D, Waring G O, Bridges W Z et al 1987 Effect of donor epithelium on corneal transplant survival. Ophthalmology 95: 803–812

Treseler P A, Sanfilippo F 1985 Humoral immunity to heterotopic corneal allografts in the rat. Transplantation 39: 193–196

Treseler P A, Foulks G N, Sanfilippo F 1984 The expression of HLA antigens by cells in the human cornea. Am J Ophthalmol 98: 763–777

Treseler P A, Foulks N, Sanfilippo F 1986 Expression of ABO blood group, haematopoietic, and other cell-specific antigens by cells in the human cornea. Cornea 4: 157–168

Troutman R C, Lawless M A 1987 Penetrating keratoplasty for keratoconus. Cornea 6: 298–305

Tuberville A W, Foster C S, Wood T O 1983 The effect of donor cornea epithelium removal on the incidence of allograft rejection reactions. Ophthalmology 90: 1351–1356

Van Horn D L, Schultz R O 1977 Corneal preservation: recent advances. Surv Ophthalmol 21: 301–312

Volker-Dieben H J, D-Amaro J, Kok-van-Alphen C C 1987 Hierarchy of prognostic factors for corneal allograft survival. Aust NZ J Ophthalmol 15: 11–18

Weiss A, Imboden J B 1987 Cell surface molecules and early events involved in human T-lymphocyte activation. Adv Immunol 41: 1–38

Williams K A, Coster D J 1989 The role of the limbus in corneal allograft rejection. Eye 3: 158–166

Williams K A, Ash J K, Coster D J 1985a Histocompatibility antigen and passenger cell content of normal and diseased human cornea. Transplantation 39: 265–269

Williams K A, Grutzmacher R D, Roussel T J et al 1985b A comparison of the effects of topical cyclosporin and topical steroid on rabbit corneal allograft rejection. Transplantation 39: 242–244

Williams K A, Sawyer M, Alfrich S J et al 1987a First report of the Australian Corneal Graft Registry. Aust NZ J Ophthalmol 15: 291–302

Williams K A, Ash J K, Mann T S et al 1987b Cells infiltrating inflamed and vascularised corneas. Transplant Proc 19: 2889–2891

Williams K A, Erickson S A, Coster D J 1987c Topical steroid, cyclosporin A, and the outcome of rat corneal allografts. Br J Ophthalmol 71: 239–242

Zimmerman T, Olson R J, Waltman S et al 1978 Transplant size and elevated intraocular pressure post-keratoplasty. Arch Ophthalmol 96: 2231–2233

4

Complications of intraocular lenses

A. D. McG. Steele

INTRODUCTION

Attitudes and practice related to intraocular lenses have undergone dramatic changes in the last ten years. The use of intraocular lenses as a routine part of the surgical management of cataract has gained widespread acceptance. This has been achieved by helpful developments of new lens styles and surgical techniques which have combined to improve the results and at the same time lower the incidence of complications which can reasonably be attributed to the intraocular lens.

Despite this welcome achievement, one needs to be constantly aware that this type of surgery does carry a complication rate, albeit a low one. These complications, which are of several different types, mean that we need an up-to-date appreciation of the situation so that appropriate clinical judgment can be exercised, patients can be correctly advised on risk/benefit ratios and further research and development can be stimulated.

This chapter will concentrate upon complications attributable to the intraocular lens rather than those attributable to the surgery. Bad surgery will always have a higher incidence of problems for which the implant should not be blamed.

COMPLICATIONS ATTRIBUTABLE TO IMPLANTS IN GENERAL

Implant surgery with any variety of lens can be followed by complications common to all varieties. There are four important instances.

Corneal endothelial decompensation

Causes

If we exclude the cases where cataract is associated with a pre-existing endothelial disorder, corneae may decompensate following intraocular lens surgery both as a result of damage sustained by the endothelium at the time of surgery and progressive damage to the endothelium following surgery (Apple et al 1984, McDonnell et al 1986, Garner 1989). The introduction of any style of intraocular lens may cause damage to the posterior surface of the cornea during manoeuvres associated with its insertion. This may occur either because of direct contact between the intraocular lens and the corneal endothelium or by direct damage caused by instruments used to assist the implantation process.

Anterior chamber lenses by virtue of the position they take up across the anterior chamber are the most likely to be brought into direct contact with the corneal endothelium during the process of introduction. Polymethyl-methacrylate (PMMA) has long been known to be responsible for direct damage to endothelial cells, should contact occur (Kaufman et al 1977). Surface modification of the PMMA may, perhaps, reduce this risk (Balyeat et al 1989). Also, all varieties of iris-supported implants other than the lobster claw lens of Worst are notoriously associated with endothelial damage during insertion because of their significantly increased antero-posterior dimensions. Of all lens styles currently in use those least likely to be associated with this problem are those designed for fixation in the posterior chamber. These are directed posteriorly across the anterior chamber and their shape is such that inadvertent contact between the lens and the corneal endothelium is unlikely. Instrumental damage, however, can still occur.

After implantation it is unlikely that posterior chamber lenses will be associated with progressive endothelial failure and this is borne out by the results of the ten years' experience we now have with their use. Pseudophakic bullous keratopathy, however, continues to be a leading indication for penetrating keratoplasty both in the USA (Robin et al 1986) and in the UK. This regrettable situation is predominantly due to the use of anterior chamber and iris-supported implants (Garner 1989), both of which can be associated with progressive endothelial damage over many years. This is caused either by peripheral irritation of the corneal endothelium adjacent to the foot of an anteriorly placed implant, or by intermittent touch between an implant and the posterior surface of the cornea. Intermittent touch can occur with any variety of anterior chamber lens and any variety of iris-supported lens. It is difficult to imagine that the simple human behavioural act of eye rubbing would not under these circumstances be associated with damage to the cornea. For iris-supported implants it is well recognized that the iris–lens diaphragm can move forwards and backwards and allow intermittent touch by this means.

Clinical course

Progressive damage to the corneal endothelium may be detected by inspection with the slit-lamp. The corneal endothelial cells may be seen to be enlarged so that the cellular mosaic becomes easily visible to the examiner without the aid of a specular microscope. These endothelial changes will be seen before the appearance of corneal oedema. When oedema does first appear it will commonly be seen to develop in an area related to the causative agent, particularly the foot of an anterior chamber lens or an anterior supporting loop of an iris-supported implant. Central corneal oedema will result in blurred vision. Initially this is usually associated with a diurnal pattern, with mistiness in the early morning which then gradually clears. The clearing time, however, becomes longer and longer until eventually the cornea fails to clear even at the end of the day. As bullae develop in the oedematous surface layers, the epithelium may become unstable and give rise to painful spontaneous erosions. By this time the vision will usually be severely impaired.

Management

The onset of early oedema related to an implant foot or haptic may prompt the surgeon to attempt to remove the implant in the hope of arresting the endothelial damage. Unfortunately, this is seldom successful as the trauma of implant removal is likely to result in immediate loss of endothelial function.

The pain of early bullous keratopathy may be satisfactorily controlled by the use of a thin soft contact lens which will protect the unstable epithelium from the abrasive effect of lid movements and exposure. If, however, pain fails to be controlled by this means or the quality of vision is so bad as to be severely affecting the patient's lifestyle, penetrating keratoplasty will be required.

When corneal grafting is required for this condition a decision needs to be made in connection with the implant in place. If the implant can reasonably be held responsible for corneal damage, e.g. with corneal oedema related to a loop or a foot or known implant mobility, then the implant must be removed. It is the author's belief that most anterior chamber and iris-supported implants fall into this category. Securely placed posterior chamber intraocular implants, however, are unlikely to be blameworthy in the same way and can usually be safely left in place. The next question to be decided is whether the implant to be removed should be replaced with another. This will depend upon the individual patient's clinical circumstances. A one-eyed patient, for example, may best be managed by corneal grafting and implant removal alone and subsequent correction of the postoperative aphakia with a spectacle lens. Other patients may be deemed suitable for management by postoperative fitting of a suitable contact lens. There will be other cases for whom neither of these options appears adequate, particularly for patients who are phakic or satisfactorily pseudophakic in the other eye. Under these circumstances an attempt should be made to replace the intraocular implant. The best lenses to use under these circumstances are some variety of open looped flexible anterior chamber lens or else a lens secured in the posterior chamber (Waring et al 1987, Van der Schaft et al 1989). In the absence of an existing capsular framework this latter option necessitates more complicated surgery including an anterior vitrectomy and scleral fixation of the intraocular lens.

Infective endophthalmitis

Any intraocular surgical procedure may be followed by the disastrous complication of infection and this naturally applies to any cataract procedure (Christy & Lall 1973). The use of an intraocular lens probably increases this risk (Bohigian & Olk 1986).

Causes

The insertion of any style of intraocular lens may be followed by this serious sight-threatening complication. The most likely cause is contamination of the implant by bacteria from the surface of the eye (Dilly & Holmes Sellors 1989) and in the vicinity of the cataract wound (Vafidis et al 1984, Griffiths et al 1989). Such contamination, of course, is more likely if the implant is placed upon the surface of the eye or anywhere near the lid margins. Inappropriate or inadvertent contact of this sort must be strenuously avoided. It is possible also that this complication is lessened by reducing the potential for bacterial adhesion to the PMMA surface by thorough rinsing with saline immediately prior to insertion.

Other causative factors associated with this complication are diabetes mellitus and the presence of active lid margin infection or lacrimal drainage obstruction. Diabetes mellitus should be brought under as close control as possible prior to cataract surgery, but even then the danger exists. Lid margin infection should be controlled before cataract surgery by the appropriate use of antibiotics. Demonstrable lacrimal obstruction, which can be occult in the elderly, may well require corrective surgery before embarking upon an elective intraocular procedure, particularly implant surgery. One rare form of infection with *Propionibacterium acnes* (Meisler et al 1986, Glenn & Wood 1988) is particularly liable to occur with bag placement of a posterior chamber lens resulting in local intraocular relative anoxia. This infection is referred to further in relation to complications of posterior chamber lenses.

Clinical course

In severe cases infective endophthalmitis may be diagnosed within the first 24 hours of surgery. Often, however, the onset of clinically detectable infection is delayed for several days. The diagnosis is usually associated with pain and inflammation in the eye but is always associated with poor vision. With severe uveitis there will frequently be a hypopyon present together with visible cellular activity within the anterior vitreous cavity.

Management

Apart from the preventative measures mentioned above, all cataract patients should be treated preoperatively with a broad-spectrum topical antibiotic. The use of subconjunctival antibiotics at the end of the surgical procedure may give a wider margin of safety.

The diagnosis of infective postoperative endophthalmitis represents an ophthalmic emergency. Patients require admission to hospital and every effort must be made to isolate the causative organism. In all cases this requires a vitreous tap procedure, best achieved by means of a pars plana approach and the use of mechanical vitrectomy equipment. Samples taken from the anterior vitreous are then spun down for the preparation of smears and culture inoculation. At the same time it is usually advisable for these severely at-risk patients to be treated by intravitreal antibiotics even before the organism has been identified. Currently, a combination of amikacin and vancomycin is advised. The patient will need intensive treatment with systemic and topical antibiotics depending upon the results of the smear culture and sensitivity. Local steroids are usually curtailed during this period as their use may promote rapid bacterial replication. Once the infection is deemed to be under control, steroids may be added to the regime in an effort to lessen the inflammatory damage to the eye.

Acute non-infective fibrinous anterior uveitis

This complication may also follow the insertion of any style of intraocular implant.

Causes

The causes are not understood. As the complication may be particularly common and severe in children who have undergone insertion of an intraocular implant (Burke et al 1989), the response may well be related to tissue immaturity resulting in an exaggeration of the normal uveitic reaction to an intraocular procedure. The complication, however, is also seen in adults and has been variously attributed to different uses of visco elastic agents or irrigation fluids. No proof for any of these, however, is forthcoming.

Clinical picture

This fibrinous uveitis is not usually detected until after the third or fourth postoperative day, although sometimes it may be seen earlier. The pupillary area and then the anterior chamber may be filled with fine fibrinous strands which will bind down the pupil and enwrap the intraocular lens. A brisk cellular response will usually be detectable in addition. Vision is impaired and there will occasionally be some associated elevation of the intraocular pressure.

Management

The treatment of this condition is by the generous application of topical steroids, e.g. dexamethasone hourly for a period of 48–72 hours. This will usually require admission to hospital for close observation because of the risk that the inflammation represents an uncommon variety of infective endophthalmitis which will be made significantly worse by intensive steroids rather than better. Gradually the fibrin will be seen to resorb, restoring freedom to the pupil, which should be kept widely dilated, so as to keep clear the visual pathway. Occasionally, a dense fibrous envelope will remain around the intraocular lens and if this does not clear spontaneously it may require surgical excision. Attempts to remove these thick fibrous envelopes by means of the YAG laser may result in a significant degree of corneal endothelial damage and glaucoma.

Chronic low-grade anterior uveitis

This complication may be seen to be associated with any variety of lens style and the complication may persist for many months after surgery.

Causes

The causative factors are not well understood, but they are presumably related to direct irritation of the anterior uveal tract by the implant itself. Only those implants which have been carefully placed and maintained postoperatively within the capsular bag can be considered to be not in direct contact with uveal tissue at some point. The points in question are the root of the iris anteriorly adjacent to the anterior chamber angle and the root of the iris posteriorly adjacent to the ciliary sulcus. For iris-supported implants, of course, the points of contact are many and may be of extensive area. PMMA, polypropylene and the soft lens materials in current use may all be seen to be associated with this complication. It is suggested that the surface coating of PMMA with heparin (Fagerholm 1989) may reduce the incidence of this complication.

Clinical picture

This problem is usually symptomless, but is detected by the observing ophthalmologist with the use of the slit-lamp. The very faintest degree of cellular activity may be detected with a very small number of circulating cells in the anterior chamber. There are seldom any keratic precipitates but some cellular precipitation on the surface of the implant is a characteristic phenomenon (Ohara 1985). Surface modification of PMMA as described above appears to be associated with fewer of these visible precipitates. Whether the underlying inflammation is also less remains speculative. Early indications that chronic low-grade uveitis may be a cause of late endothelial failure (Rao et al 1981) do no yet seem to have proved accurate.

Management

In this connection iris-supported implants should be avoided as they are nearly always associated with some degree of detectable chronic anterior uveitis, although in most cases there do not appear to be any clinical consequences. Anterior chamber lenses when their use is deemed necessary for the patient's best management must be seen to be well fitting to avoid irritation caused by mobility of the foot or the stress of an overlong lens. Posterior chamber lenses should be placed 'in the bag' wherever possible in order to avoid uveal contact. The only sure way of ensuring no late partial escape from the capsular bag as a result of capsular splitting is to use an implant which fits the bag's dimensions preceded by management of the anterior capsule by capsulorhexis. This technique provides a very strong capsular edge which is not prone to late stress rupture. Because of its known tendency to biodegradation the use of polypropylene supporting haptics even in the posterior chamber should probably be discontinued, particularly for lenses inserted into younger patients. Where precipitates on the lens surface interfere with vision or represent an unacceptable degree of anterior chamber activity local steroid medication should be used for as long as is necessary to overcome the problem at a clinical level. It is probable that some subclinical uveitic activity may continue indefinitely.

COMPLICATIONS SPECIFICALLY RELATED TO LENS STYLES OR PLACEMENT

Anterior chamber lenses

All forms of anterior chamber lens are supported by the structures of the chamber angle. The complications related to their use can reasonably be attributed to their proximity to the adjacent corneal endothelium and to direct damage to the angle of the anterior chamber itself.

Rigid anterior chamber intraocular lenses

Size problems. The chief problem with the concept of these lenses is the difficulty of obtaining a perfect fit – neither too loose nor too tight. Loose intraocular implants are too short and can always be seen to be mobile. On consecutive examinations they may be recorded as rotating in the chamber angle, changing their orientation by as much as 90° between visits. Such implants are a hazard to the corneal endothelium and to the chamber angle structures and when detected should always be removed and replaced. Implants which fit securely do so by applying constant pressure to the angle structures responsible for their support. This invariably gives rise to pain or tenderness to touch. This tenderness may serve to protect the patient, who is deterred from eye rubbing with its consequent risks of endothelial damage, but it can also be a distressing symptom. Although such implants are less likely to be associated with progressive corneal endothelial damage they are more likely to be associated with progressive damage to the iris, usually revealed as a progressive ovaling of the pupil in the same axis as the intraocular lens. This ovaling of the pupil is probably attributable to relative ischaemia produced by the pressure of the implant feet.

Implants which are too long cause constant pain as well as progressive oval distortion of the pupil. In addition they will in some cases cause a cyclodialysis. This in turn leads to instability of the lens with greatly increased risk of damage to the cornea.

Uveitis, glaucoma, hyphaema ('UGH') syndrome. The classical UGH syndrome was first described in relation to rigid anterior chamber lenses (Ellingson 1977). The causative factor was found to be defective manufacture, which left rough edges on the feet of the implant, giving rise to the inflammation and vascular damage which produced the triad of uveitis, glaucoma and hyphaema. The syndrome, however, has not disappeared with the correction of the manufacturing defect and has been associated with most forms of anterior chamber intraocular lens styles from time to time. When this triad of problems does arise it probably requires the removal of the offending implant.

Chronic glaucoma. Even in the absence of clinical uveitis some of these patients with rigid anterior chamber lenses will develop glaucoma because of angle recession (Garner 1989) or chronic angle closure which may be slowly but relentlessly progressive. Unfortunately, removal of the implant will not alleviate this problem which therefore requires medical and possibly hazardous surgical management. Unfortunately, in most cases, the use of an anterior chamber intraocular lens has been associated with either intracapsular cataract extraction or an unsuccessful attempt at extracapsular cataract extraction. Under these circumstances the surgical management of ensuing chronic glaucoma is much more difficult than is experienced after successful extracapsular cataract extraction. The latter successfully excludes the vitreous base from interfering with the filtration process.

Flexible anterior chamber intraocular lenses

These were designed to overcome problems of good fit. Initially, such implants were used 40 years ago and were associated with a disastrously high incidence of corneal disorders. More modern styles included those with both open and closed loops although the closed loop styles have almost entirely disappeared from the lens market. They were associated with anterior vaulting and an increased risk of damage to the corneal endothelium as well as with erosion of the structures of the angle of the anterior chamber and a high incidence of glaucoma (Reidy et al 1985, Smith et al 1987).

Several attempts have been made to design an anterior chamber lens supported by flexible haptics of such a design that one size of implant would fit all anterior chambers. This concept so far has failed to work. One lens of this type, used in particular by Barraquer in the 1950s in Spain, resulted in many cases of subsequent corneal endothelial decompensation. This particular experience later led to the long delayed acceptance in Spain of modern intraocular lens progress, a problem now happily overcome.

Another style of flexible open looped implant designed to fit all anterior chambers was produced by Shepherd in the USA. Although not approved by the FDA for regular use in the USA and never used, so far as the author is aware, in the UK, these implants have been made available in various centres elsewhere around the world. Unfortunately, their construction does not fulfil the requirements of their original design. The flexible haptics are prone to lose their memory so that the implants become loose within the anterior chamber and can produce rapid endothelial destruction.

The lens now in most widespread use in the anterior chamber is a semi-flexible open-loop style made of PMMA originally designed by Kelman and incorporating four separate points of fixation. The type of lens appears to be associated with a lower incidence of problems, although the inherent disadvantages of this form of placement continue to apply.

Iris-supported intraocular lenses

The development of these lenses particularly by Binkhorst was a crucial step in the development of surgery now in popular practice. The incidence of late complications, however, particularly corneal endothelial failure (Apple et al 1984, Garner 1989), has seen their demise. This particular complication has already been considered in some detail in the earlier part of this chapter, together with its management. It is the author's opinion that iris-supported implants should almost always be removed if penetrating keratoplasty is required. This will almost certainly need an associated anterior vitrectomy and the patient will then be best managed by the insertion of a posterior chamber lens using scleral fixation. Alternatively, an anterior chamber lens may be used if a semi-flexible variety, providing that the angle of the anterior chamber can be seen to be normal and the patient free of any history of raised intraocular pressure.

Apart from this complication, iris-supported intraocular lenses lead to small immobile pupils, iris sphincter erosion and pigment dispersion. An increased incidence of chronic low-grade uveitis and the probable association of cystoid macular oedema is now generally accepted. Because of these connections with sight-threatening complications iris-supported implants have now been abandoned by most surgeons in favour of posterior chamber lenses.

Posterior chamber intraocular lenses

Optically and physiologically the posterior chamber is the logical site for a replacement of the natural lens. Its greatest advantage is that it is as far away as possible from the corneal endothelium and it is therefore expected that routine posterior chamber placement of intraocular implants will lead to a significant fall in the incidence of late-onset pseudophakic bullous keratopathy. In cases where this complication does arise, the endothelial damage has probably been sustained at the time of the surgery. Where penetrating keratoplasty is required these lenses may usually safely be left in situ. Other complications which may arise are as follows.

Capsule opacification

Extracapsular cataract surgery which leaves an intact posterior capsule carries the inevitable risk of eventual capsule opacification.

Causes. Capsule opacification is the result of a combination of fibrosis and the migration of new lens fibres produced by the germinal epithelium at the capsule periphery. While these factors are not a direct consequence of intraocular lens implantation the progress of capsular opacification can certainly be modified by implant design. A laser ridge at the posterior periphery of the lens optic may impede migration of fibroblasts and new lens fibres across the posterior capsule by presenting a barrier between the laser ridge and the stretched posterior capsule. There is a further theoretical advantage of such a ridge in that it will hold the stretched posterior capsule away from the posterior surface of the implant, a help for safer laser capsulotomy. It would appear, however, that a more effective barrier to capsular opacification in the visual area is provided by the direct apposition of the steeper convex posterior surface of the implant directly applied to the capsule itself. Most intraocular lenses for the posterior chamber currently available have a biconvex profile with the steeper curvature posteriorly. Laser ridges are being abandoned.

Clinical features. Capsular opacification is associated with loss of vision. In the early stages this may only be appreciated as a loss of contrast sensitivity or a visual impairment under reduced illumination. As the opacification proceeds, however, visual acuity will fall and if left untreated the vision may become seriously impaired.

Clinical management. The simplest form of management is by neodymium–YAG laser posterior capsulotomy. Where this form of treatment is not available, surgical capsulotomy will be required and this is probably best achieved via the pars plana. Attempts have been made to inhibit the growth of fibrous tissue and the replication of lens fibres by the use of cryo treatment to the capsule after aspiration of the peripheral cortex or by the transient application of chemical toxic agents. It is probable that the best of these preventative techniques is the careful vacuuming of remaining germinal epithelial cells from the peripheral capsule after complete removal of the cortical material.

Intraocular lens displacement

Prior to the regular inclusion of a 10–15° angulation between the lens haptics and optical zone, forward movement of the implant could be associated with pupil capture leading to a cat-eye deformity of the pupil. If detected early this can usually be reversed by dilating the pupil, posturing the patient and then constricting the pupil so that it comes down in front of the implant. If not detected early, however, the pupil capture leads to the development of synechiae and irreversibility. Although the vision is seldom affected there is a greatly increased risk of low-grade chronic uveitis. Since the use of uniplanar posterior chamber lenses has been abandoned this complication has become less common. Late rupture of the posterior capsule or dehiscence of the lens zonule may result in intraocular lens instability so that one or both haptics may become displaced into the posterior vitreous cavity. Should a lens become totally dislocated it is probably best left alone, but where one haptic only becomes displaced surgical correction should be attempted. This may be achieved by a small incision in the pars plana through which the displaced haptic can be retrieved and sutured to the inner lip of the scleral wound.

More commonly, posterior chamber implants can become displaced in the plane of the implant and will lead to decentration.

Decentration

Causes. Most commonly this will occur where one haptic is within the lens capsule and the other is not. Partial dehiscence of the lens zonule can produce a similar effect. In implants using haptics of extruded PMMA or polypropylene the inbuilt memory for the proper curvature of the haptic may be lost if a deformity is permitted to persist for any length of time.

Clinical picture. Decentration is not usually associated with loss of visual acuity unless the implant is very severely displaced. Optical aberrations are more common when optic edge structures including the rim of the lens, the root of a haptic or a positioning hole become visible within the pupillary aperture (Apple et al 1987, Ohara & Abe 1989, Obstbaum & To 1989). These aberrations are particularly troublesome at night and when viewing illuminated objects such as lamps, a television screen, street lights and vehicle headlights. These can give rise to tiresome streaks and multiple images which may be disabling, in which case, corrective surgery will usually be required.

Clinical management. The use of implants with larger optical areas which do not include positioning holes has proved to be the best preventative measure for the abolition of symptoms associated with minor degrees of decentration. In addition, the regular use of bag placement for posterior chamber implants is helpful, but this can only be relied upon to be a long-term placement if the anterior capsule has been managed by capsulorhexis. Other forms of anterior capsule management, though assisting bag placement at the time of surgery, can all be associated with late capsule splitting and the escape of one haptic from the bag into the ciliary sulcus. Where decentration gives rise to troublesome symptoms these may be eliminated by the use of a weak miotic agent, e.g. pilocarpine 0.5%, to be used before night driving. Where this measure is unacceptable or fails to correct the problem, the decentration will need to be surgically corrected. Where the haptic design has not included kinks or knobs on the end of the haptic the implant may be rotated so that the haptics become free of the capsule and will locate in the ciliary sulcus. Providing no loss of memory of curvature has occurred the decentration will be seen to be corrected. Where this measure fails, however, the implant will need to be removed. Haptics that cannot be withdrawn need to be divided with scissors and the remaining fragments left in situ. A new implant is then inserted with the haptic supported by the ciliary sulcus.

Anisometropia

Causes. Occasionally, preoperative biometry may fail to predict accurately the power of the implant required so that the patient is left with a degree of intolerable anisometropia.

Clinical picture. Under these circumstances the patient's optical problems may give rise to aniseikonia or spatial aberrations.

Clinical management. Attempts to fit patients with correcting glasses are usually unsuccessful. An attempt may be made to fit one or other of the eyes with a correcting contact lens. Should this measure fail the only other solution is for the surgeon to re-operate and exchange the offending implant for one of the necessary power. This procedure, however, does carry some risk of damage to the posterior capsule, as well as pigment dispersion and transient secondary glaucoma.

Endophthalmitis

Although the subject of postoperative infection was discussed at the beginning of this chapter, bag-placed intraocular lenses can be associated with an unusual form of intracapsular endophthalmitis due to *Propionibacterium acnes* (Meisler et al 1986, Glenn & Wood 1988).

Causes. This infective agent is a skin and lid commensal and gains its access to the eye by adherence to the intraocular implant at the time of insertion. The relatively anoxic conditions within the implant-filled capsular bag are ideal for replication of this organism.

Clinical picture. This form of infection gives rise to an apparent low-grade chronic uveitis which is suppressed by steroid and antibiotic medication but which readily recurs when the treatment is withdrawn. This process may persist for many months. The diagnosis may be established by culture of the organism following examination of the fluid contents of the capsular bag. Where this complication cannot be satisfactorily controlled by topical antibiotics and steroids, the implant may have to be removed.

Iris chafing syndrome (Masket 1986)

Cause. This is a rare complication of posterior chamber lens implantation and is not usually seen until some years after the implant surgery. The cause is attributed to the direct irritation of a blood vessel in the iris or the ciliary sulcus by contact with one of the lens haptics, especially haptics made of polypropylene (Hakin et al 1989).

Clinical picture. This complication is characterized by 'white outs' of the vision. These are usually transient and are due to the sudden release of minute amounts of blood into the aqueous from the damaged vessel. Examination reveals iris transillumination defects, pigment dispersion and glaucoma as well as the presence of red blood corpuscles in the aqueous fluid (Johnson et al 1984).

Clinical management. These symptoms can be controlled by keeping the pupil widely dilated in the hope that this will prevent the direct contact causing the problem. Should this fail the intraocular implant may need to be removed and replaced. The regular use of bag placement of intraocular implants in the posterior chamber, however, should significantly reduce the likelihood of this late complication.

Problems associated with soft intraocular lens materials

Experimentation continues with intraocular lens materials other than polymethylmethacrylate and two in particular have been tried, namely silicone and polyhema, the same materials as are used in soft contact lenses. Both these materials have been shown to be biologically inert and their hydrophilic surface properties make them well suited to intraocular usage. Most of the problems with these lenses have arisen because of the difficulties connected with their supporting architecture (Condon et al 1989, Bucher et al 1989). Attempts to make these lenses suitable for bag placement have been followed by an inability for the lens material to resist the contracting forces of a shrinking capsule. This has led to distortion and displacement of the implant. In some cases late tearing of the posterior capsule has resulted in the sudden displacement of the implant into the vitreous cavity and in this instance the fault is clearly related to the implant itself. The growing demand for small incision surgery, however, continues to lead developers to find an answer to these problems (Neumann & Cobb 1989) and the commonest solution so far is the development of a soft lens optic which can be folded, supported by semi-flexible polypropylene haptics. Smaller one-piece polyhema intraocular implants are also undergoing trial with the hope that they will not give rise to the same problems of posterior capsular splitting if they are secured within the capsular bag.

Problems associated with bi- or multifocal intraocular implants

More recent still is the development of multifocal or bifocal posterior chamber implants. These are designed to overcome the disadvantages of fixed focus lenses so that a patient may enjoy good uncorrected vision both for distance and for near. Apart from the difficulties of achieving just the right postoperative refractive situation, the major disadvantage of this form of implant appears to be the loss of contrast sensitivity at high frequencies. This is particularly noticeable to patients who have a unifocal intraocular implant in one eye and a bifocal or multifocal implant in the other. The constant presence of some degree of defocused light falling upon the retina at all fixation distances does give rise to a degree of ineradicable blur. It would appear that the only way to overcome this difficulty is the production of a lens which will change shape and power for varying focusing distances. Such a concept is unlikely to be beyond human ingenuity.

SUMMARY

Modern cataract surgery with the insertion of posterior chamber intraocular lenses carries an astonishingly high success rate and a very pleasingly low level of complication. The use of anterior chamber lenses should be regarded as a second-best option to be employed only when posterior chamber implantation is deemed either unsafe or impracticable. Posterior chamber lenses should be secured within the capsular bag wherever possible to minimize the risk of complications.

REFERENCES

Apple D J, Mamalis N, Loftfield K et al 1984 Complications of intraocular lenses: an historical and histopathological review. Surv Ophthalmol 29: 1–54
Apple D J, Lichtenstein S B, Heerlein K et al 1987 Visual aberrations caused by optic components of posterior chamber intraocular lenses. J Cataract Refract Surg 13: 431–435
Balyeat H D, Nordquist R E, Lerner M P et al 1989 Comparison of endothelial damage produced by control and surface modified poly(methylmethacrylate) intraocular lenses. J Cataract Refract Surg 15: 491–494
Bohigian G M, Olk R J 1986 Factors associated with a poor visual result in endophthalmitis. Am J Ophthalmol 101: 332–341
Bucher P J M, Schimmelpfennig B, Faggioni R 1989 One year follow-up of IOGEL intraocular lenses with ciliary sulcus fixation. J Cataract Refract Surg 15: 635–639
Burke J P, Willshaw H E, Young J D H 1989 Intraocular lens implants for uniocular cataracts in childhood. Br J Ophthalmol 73: 860–864
Christy N E, Lall P 1973 Postoperative endophthalmitis following cataract surgery: effects of subconjunctival antibiotics and other factors. Arch Ophthalmol 90: 361–366
Condon P I, Barrett G D, Kinsella M 1989 Results of the intercapsular technique with the IOGEL lens. J Cataract Refract Surg 15: 495–503
Dilly P N, Holmes Sellors P J 1989 Bacterial adhesion to intraocular lenses. J Cataract Refract Surg 15: 317–320
Ellingson F T 1977 Complications with the Choyce Mark VII anterior chamber lens implant (uveitis–glaucoma–hyphaema). J Am Intraocular Implant Soc 3: 199–206
Fagerholm P, Bjorklund H, Holmberg A et al 1989 Heparin surface modified intraocular lenses implanted in the monkey eye. J Cataract Refract Surg 15: 485–490
Garner A 1989 Complications of prosthetic intraocular lens implantation: a histopathological study. Br J Ophthalmol 73: 940–945
Glenn A M, Wood C M 1988 Propionibacterium acnes. Br Med J 297: 201–202
Griffiths P G, Elliott T S J, McTaggart L 1989 Adherence of staphylococcus epidermidis to

intraocular lenses. Br J Ophthalmol 73: 402–406

Hakin K, Batterbury M, Hawksworth N et al 1989 Anterior tucking of the iris caused by posterior chamber lenses with polypropylene loops. J Cataract Refract Surg 15: 640–643

Johnson S H, Kratz R P, Olson P F 1984 Iris transillumination defects and microhyphema syndrome. J Am Intraocular Implant Soc 10: 425–428

Kaufman H E, Katz J, Valenti J et al 1977 Corneal endothelium damage with intraocular lenses: contact adhesion between surgical materials and tissue. Science 198: 525–527

Masket S 1986 Pseudophakic posterior iris chafing syndrome. J Cataract Refract Surg 12: 252–256

McDonnell P J, Green W R, Champion R 1986 Pathologic changes in pseudophakia. Semin Ophthalmol 1: 80–103

Meisler D M, Palestine A G, Vastine D W et al 1986 Chronic *Propionibacterium* endophthalmitis after extracapsular cataract extraction and intraocular lens implantation. Am J Ophthalmol 102: 733–739

Neumann A C, Cobb B 1989 Advantages and limitations of current soft intraocular lenses. J Cataract Refract Surg 15: 257–263

Obstbaum S A, To K 1989 Posterior chamber intraocular lens dislocations and malpositions. Aust NZ J Ophthalmol 17: 265–271

Ohara K 1985 Biomicroscopy of surface deposits resembling foreign-body giant cells on implanted intraocular lenses. Am J Ophthalmol 99: 304–311

Ohara K, Abe K 1989 Role of positioning holes in intraocular lens glare. J Cataract Refract Surg 15: 647–653

Rao G N, Stevens R E, Harris J K, Aquavella J V 1981 Long term changes in corneal endothelium following intraocular lens implantation. Ophthalmology 88: 386–397

Reidy J J, Apple D J, Googe J M et al 1985 An analysis of semiflexible closed loop anterior chamber intraocular lenses. J Am Intraocular Implant Soc 11: 344–352

Robin J B, Gindi J J, Koh K et al 1986 An update of the indications for penetrating keratoplasty 1979 through 1983. Arch Ophthalmol 104: 87–89

Smith P W, Wong S K, Stark W J et al 1987 Complications of semiflexible closed loop anterior chamber intraocular lenses. Arch Ophthalmol 105: 52–57

Vafidis G C, Marsh R J, Stacey A R 1984 Bacterial contamination of intraocular lens surgery. Br J Ophthalmol 68: 520–523

van der Schaft T L, van Rij G, Renardell de Lavalette J G C et al 1989 Results of penetrating keratoplasty for pseudophakic bullous keratopathy with the exchange of an intraocular lens. Br J Ophthalmol 73: 704–708

Waring G O, Stulting R D, Street D 1987 Penetrating keratoplasty for pseudophakic corneal edema with exchange of intraocular lenses. Arch Ophthalmol 105: 58–62

5

Medical versus surgical treatment of primary open angle glaucoma

J. L. Jay

INTRODUCTION

Despite scepticism from some authorities, it is generally agreed that treatment for glaucoma is beneficial. In primary open angle glaucoma, all forms of therapy aim to reduce an intraocular pressure which has either caused damage to the ganglion cells at the optic nerve head, with resultant loss of visual field, or is perceived to have a significant risk of causing damage in the future.

EFFECT OF THERAPY ON INTRAOCULAR PRESSURE

All three commonly used forms of therapy – topical or systemic drugs, argon laser trabeculoplasty and drainage surgery – lower intraocular pressure in most cases. The reduction is proportional to the initial level of pressure. Drainage surgery is the most effective; trabeculectomy reduces the pressure to the physiological range, irrespective of the level of pressure before treatment (Jay & Murray 1980). Comparative trials indicate that the three methods of treatment are not equally effective. Smith (1972) showed the greater effectiveness of drainage surgery over medical therapy in lowering intraocular pressure. This has been confirmed by Migdal & Hitchings (1986), who also found that the effect of argon laser trabeculoplasty lay between the less effective medical therapy and the more effective surgery. However, Tuulonen et al (1989) found argon laser trabeculoplasty no more effective than medical therapy in lowering intraocular pressure. Jay & Murray (1988) showed that even in the 68% of cases still judged to be controlled by medical therapy at one year after diagnosis the mean intraocular pressure was 21 mmHg. This was significantly higher than the mean of 15 mmHg after trabeculectomy in the same series.

The diurnal variation in intraocular pressure is almost eliminated by trabeculectomy, reduced by argon laser trabeculoplasty, and little altered by medical therapy (Migdal & Hitchings 1986). It is therefore interesting that the pathological rise in intraocular pressure during the supine provocative test remains even after successful trabeculectomy (Parsley et al 1987).

75

LEVEL OF INTRAOCULAR PRESSURE AND LOSS OF VISUAL FIELD

There is a variable relationship between intraocular pressure and loss of visual field, ranging from ocular hypertension with no loss of field to low-tension glaucoma with advanced field loss and little or no detectable elevation of intraocular pressure. There is, however, a link. The risk of development of visual field defects in ocular hypertension increases with higher intraocular pressures, especially above 30 mmHg. In established glaucoma receiving treatment, eyes with pressures below 18 mmHg were found to have half the annual rate of deterioration of mean retinal sensitivity of eyes with intraocular pressure above 18 mmHg (Crick et al 1989). Jay & Allen (1989) found that at diagnosis and before treatment eyes with mild relative visual field defects had significantly lower pressures than those with absolute scotomas, but that increasing area of absolute scotoma was not associated with progressively higher pressure. In patients with low-tension glaucoma, the eye with the worse visual field loss tends to have the higher intraocular pressure (Cartwright & Anderson 1988, Crichton et al 1989). Therefore, there is now enough evidence to associate higher intraocular pressure with greater visual field damage in most cases. Is the raised intraocular pressure the cause of the field loss? We must examine the evidence that lowering intraocular pressure improves visual field survival.

The effect of lowering intraocular pressure on visual field survival

There have been few comparative trials of treatment versus no treatment, but in 1966 Becker & Morton demonstrated the value of adrenaline eye drops in reducing the risk of visual field loss in ocular hypertension. The benefit was greatest where the untreated pressure was higher than 24 mmHg. More recently, Epstein et al (1989) compared timolol therapy with no therapy in ocular hypertension with pressures between 22 and 28 mmHg. They found that treatment lowered the risk of progressive disc cupping and field loss. Most of the patients in the treatment group who showed deterioration had not been using treatment reliably. Holmin et al (1988) were unable to detect any difference in visual field progression in treated and untreated groups, but in their study the mean pressure difference between the groups was small and treatment compliance seemed uncertain.

There is evidence that eyes with optic nerve damage caused by glaucoma require an intraocular pressure well below the arbitrary top level of normal of 20–22 mmHg if further field loss is to be avoided. Freyler & Menapace (1988) found that treated eyes becoming blind from glaucoma had higher intraocular pressure than fellow eyes which retained vision. Those with pressure less than 17 mmHg did better than those higher in the normal range. This confirmed a study by Odberg (1987), where the best prognosis in advanced glaucoma was associated with a pressure less than 15 mmHg. Fifty eight per cent of the eyes with pressure less than 15 mmHg (and in most cases this had been achieved by drainage surgery) had stable visual fields, compared with 29% of the whole study population. Sponsel (1989) dismisses the importance of intraocular pressure as a screening test, which is a result of fluctuation in pressure making a single normal reading unreliable. He also claims that reduction of intraocular pressure does not correlate with visual field survival. This may indicate that the mean pressure of about 21 mmHg (see above) achieved by apparently satisfactory medical therapy may be insufficient when compared with the lower mean pressure of 15 mmHg after trabeculectomy. Increased vulnerability to a pressure in the high normal range may be explained by structural changes in the lamina cribrosa which make the ganglion cell axons progressively more susceptible to pressure damage as glaucomatous optic atrophy advances. For example, Miller & Quigley (1988) have suggested that elongation of the pores of the lamina in eyes with more advanced damage may lower the threshold for nerve fibre atrophy. Furthermore, the persisting diurnal variation in pressure on medical treatment may be damaging. Although the eyes which continue to lose visual field after trabeculectomy (Kidd & O'Connor 1985) do not have a mean intraocular pressure different from those which remain stable, they do seem to have a more variable pressure (Werner et al 1977).

Trabeculectomy at diagnosis provides significant protection of visual field when compared with eyes given an initial trial of medical treatment. The extra deterioration with the latter method occurs during the unsuccessful attempt at medical control (Jay & Murray 1988, Jay & Allen 1989). It is possible that this arises partly from poor compliance with medical therapy. If so, it strengthens the argument that the difference is related to more successful lowering of pressure after trabeculectomy. In Smith's study (Smith 1972, 1986) the inconclusive results for difference in visual field may be attributed to the trial design, which did not selectively examine the changes in field in the first and second years after diagnosis. It was in this period that Jay & Allen (1989) found the main benefit from early surgery. Once the eyes which were poorly controlled medically had been identified and subjected to trabeculectomy, the group visual field deterioration was much slower and similar to that of the group which had early surgery (Fig. 5.1).

In low-tension glaucoma, de Jong et al (1989) found that filtering operations were significantly better for stabilizing visual field loss than continuing medical therapy. Operation also achieved lower intraocular pressure and less diurnal variation.

METHODS OF TREATMENT

Medical therapy, argon laser trabeculoplasty and trabeculectomy are progressively more effective in lowering intraocular pressure. Nevertheless, choice of therapy for different stages of glaucoma depends on a more critical awareness of the comparative benefits and risks of each.

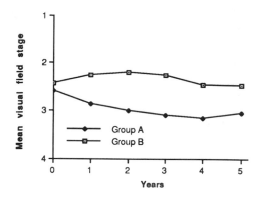

Fig. 5.1 The group mean visual field stage at each year of follow-up for eyes treated conventionally (group A) and eyes treated by early trabeculectomy (group B). During the first two years group A deteriorated relative to group B. Thereafter, most of the cases in group A which could not be controlled medically had been identified and had trabeculectomy. The subsequent performance of the groups is similar. (Reproduced with permission from Jay & Allen 1989.)

Medical therapy

Eye drops have conventionally been considered safer than surgical operation, although it is well recognized that the patient may fail to take them as prescribed. Using monitored eye drop containers which indicated the true pattern of use of treatment, Kass et al (1986b) found that for pilocarpine only 76% of the prescribed treatment was taken. Six per cent of patients took less than 6% of therapy; 45% of patients had at least one day of no treatment. Compliance was much higher in the 24 hours before a visit to the doctor. Compliance with timolol was found to be little better. Only 83% of doses were used and the equivalent of one week's treatment per month was missed by 26% of patients (Kass et al 1987). In addition, they found 12.7% of patients used extra doses which might increase the risk of systemic side effects. It was impossible to identify accurately by other means the patients who did not use treatment correctly (Kass et al 1986a). In some countries and in some social circumstances long-term supply or supervision of medical therapy is not possible and here the option of early surgery has always been popular. Drug side effects are common, often limit treatment and may be life threatening, especially with beta-blockers or carbonic anhydrase inhibitors. For example, four fatalities linked to beta-blocker eye drops were reported to the Committee of Safety of Medicine in the UK up to June 1990 (CSM 1990).

Less obvious disadvantages of long-term medical therapy have recently been identified. Tauber et al (1989), reviewing 111 patients with ocular cicatricial pemphigoid, found that 26% had glaucoma. Nearly all of these had advanced glaucoma with a history of prolonged use of medication for an average 11 years before the diagnosis of pemphigoid. They also showed significantly more conjunctival injection than those with pemphigoid alone. This observation is supported by the finding of an increased amount of inflammatory cells in conjunctival biopsies from eyes on long-term medical therapy when compared with specimens from eyes treated by early trabeculectomy (Sherwood et al 1989). In a study of eyes with encapsulated filtering blebs, Richter et al (1988) reported that this complication was more commonly associated with prolonged beta-blocker therapy. Thomas & Jay (1988) similarly found that a rise in pressure with topical steroids following trabeculectomy was more common in eyes which had prior medical therapy than those without. Indeed, these two causes of early postoperative pressure rise may be the same (see below).

Perhaps the greatest risk associated with medical therapy is the loss of visual field which occurs during unsuccessful attempts to establish medical control (Jay & Murray 1988, Jay & Allen 1989). Even after initial satisfactory medical control, many eyes show gradually increasing pressure in later years while on the same therapy. This is more likely to be caused by progression of the disease than by treatment wearing off (Chauhan et al 1989).

Argon laser trabeculoplasty

The current method was introduced by Wise & Witter (1979) and at first used in the hope of avoiding drainage surgery in eyes uncontrolled by maximum medical therapy. The success in lowering intraocular pressure was rapidly confirmed by many authors, but it was found to delay rather than avoid surgical operation (Gilbert et al 1986). It is associated with significant risks (Hoskins et al 1983). For example, it may provoke dangerous elevation of intraocular pressure and loss of visual field if excessive power is applied or if 360° of the angle is treated at one time. It is safer to treat 90° or 180° at one application and to reduce the risk of acute pressure rise by pre-treatment with oral carbonic anhydrase inhibitors or beta-blocker or aproclonidine eye drops. If the patient is already on maximum medical therapy then adequate pre-treatment may be difficult without resorting to osmotic agents. Its effectiveness depends on the experience and skill of the operator (Khan et al 1986). The characteristics of the patient also influence the response to treatment. Eyes with pseudoexfoliation, pigmented meshwork or lower pre-treatment pressure levels are more likely to respond, especially in patients over 60 years of age (Ticho & Nescher 1989).

Although argon laser trabeculoplasty is initially successful in about 75% of cases, and that figure varies depending on how success is defined, it becomes gradually less effective with time. In the author's experience, the loss of effect can produce a sudden and dramatic rise in pressure. Between 5% and 10% of cases escape from control each year of follow-up (Lehmann & Faggioni 1986, Moulin et al 1987, Wise 1987, Fink et al 1988, Lund & Zink 1988). Schwartz et al (1985) found the temporary effect of treatment more marked in black patients, where the median time for the intraocular pressure to rise over 21 mmHg was 12 months, compared with 60 months for white patients. Where loss of control has occurred after initially successful treatment of up to

180° of the angle, re-treatment of the second 180° is effective (Rouhiainen & Terasvirta 1988).

Much less effect can be obtained by re-treating after initially successful 360° therapy. Using as criterion of success a reduction of merely 3 mmHg, Richter et al (1987) found only 33% of such re-treatments effective at one year. This is similar to the 38% re-treatment success with mean pressure reduction of 10.2 mmHg reported by Brown et al (1985), who warned of a serious risk of marked rise in pressure after re-treatment often needing urgent operation. Such marginal results are not worthwhile. Re-treatment will probably only delay control and risk of further loss of visual field.

Current interest in argon laser trabeculoplasty has moved from its use as a means of avoiding surgery in cases escaping from medical control to direct comparison with medical therapy as a first line of treatment in newly diagnosed cases. If effective, it should remove the worry about compliance with medical therapy, but the high rate of escape from control will require close supervision after laser trabeculoplasty. In a retrospective comparison of primary argon laser trabeculoplasty with primary medical therapy, Tuulonen et al (1987) found 50% of laser-treated eyes with pressures less than 22 mmHg at five years compared with only 22% of eyes treated medically. Although the area of the neuroretinal rim of the optic disc was better preserved in the laser-treated group, there was no detectable difference in the visual field between the groups. A subsequent randomized prospective study by the same group (Tuulonen et al 1989) showed, after one year of follow-up, no statistical difference between the two treatments for visual field, corrected neuroretinal rim area or intraocular pressure. Therefore, it seems there is little to choose between primary laser therapy and primary medical therapy.

Laser trabeculoplasty may affect the outcome of later drainage surgery. Richter et al (1988) found encapsulated filtering blebs in 15.4% of eyes which had prior argon laser trabeculoplasty and 4.7% of those which had not. If, as now seems likely, the effectiveness of laser trabeculoplasty is broadly equivalent to medical therapy, the more radical comparison is between either of these treatments and drainage surgery.

Trabeculectomy

Surgery to create a deliberate scleral fistula for aqueous humour to drain to the subconjunctival space was introduced by Lagrange in 1906 and there have been many subsequent variations. Excessively free drainage of aqueous in the early postoperative period caused unpleasant complications and usually restricted these operations to cases where the pressure could not be controlled medically.

The operations of trabeculectomy (Cairns 1968, Watson 1970) and of goniotrephination under a scleral flap (Fronimopoulos et al 1970) allowed more controlled drainage of aqueous by guarding the fistula with an intact flap of partial-thickness sclera. This modification made drainage operations safer and did not seem to reduce the probability of controlling the intraocular pressure. This last point has been studied by many authors, who do not always agree, but Parrish & Folberg (1989) provide an extensive review of studies comparing partial and full-thickness drainage operations and conclude that they are equally effective in lowering intraocular pressure. Varying the size and site of the fistula does not affect the final intraocular pressure (Duzanec & Krieglstein 1981, Osusky 1986). However, the use of topical steroids in the postoperative period enhances the chance of successful control (Starita et al 1985). The same regime of postoperative steroid drops may evoke a transient rise of pressure after trabeculectomy (Thomas & Jay 1988) and this must not be confused with failure of the operation. The 23% of eyes which showed this steroid-induced pressure rise had established drainage blebs, and it is possible that the early postoperative elevated pressure in the presence of a bleb, described by some authors as 'high bleb phase' or 'encapsulated' drainage blebs, may be a misinterpretation of the steroid response (Richter et al 1988). These are also temporary and occur in a similar proportion of eyes as the steroid-induced rise (Scott & Quigley 1988, Shingleton et al 1990).

The lower rate of complications after trabeculectomy compared with full-thickness drainage operations has caused many surgeons to re-examine the indications for surgical intervention. At present, they are far from uniform (Wilke & Storr-Paulsen 1986) and in the past the popularity of surgical rather than medical control has fluctuated. Boyd (1955) described a trend to early surgical treatment in Oxford during the Second World War because there were fears of difficulty in providing adequate supervision of long-term medical treatment. Only a few years later, the situation had reversed and he stated: 'Ocular tensions up to 35 mmHg and even higher under miotics are not now an indication for immediate operation. Even decreasing fields are not necessarily an indication for operation.' He compared cases treated either surgically or medically in these different periods, and found that cases treated medically had visual field deterioration less often. He excluded, however, cases which had uncontrolled pressure. This, with other exclusions and the retrospective nature of the study, makes his conclusions unconvincing. Furthermore, many authors have published series where surgical operation has controlled both intraocular pressure and visual field loss where both were previously uncontrolled. Smith (1986) has reported on a long-term follow-up of his series. This confirmed the lower intraocular pressure after drainage surgery compared with medical therapy and found little difference in visual field outcome. The analysis required a redistribution of the original random group allocation which made the study essentially retrospective. He was also unable to compare differences in the first few years of therapy.

The Glasgow trial of early trabeculectomy versus conventional management has provided useful information on the relative effects of medical and surgical treatment on visual field survival and gives a rational basis for the timing of trabeculectomy (Jay 1983, Jay & Murray 1988, Jay & Allen 1989). This study has been running for over nine years. It is a multicentre prospective randomized trial of management of newly diagnosed cases of primary open angle glaucoma with untreated intraocular pressure greater than 25 mmHg and glaucomatous visual field defects. Eyes with all stages of field loss were studied. They varied from having mild relative scotomas in the arcuate area outside 10° of fixation, to absolute scotomas within 5° of fixation in all quadrants. One group had trabeculectomy at diagnosis followed where necessary by medical therapy. The other group had a trial of up to three different medications and had trabeculectomy where the maximum tolerated treatment was unsuccessful in controlling intraocular pressure or visual field.

The operations were performed by surgeons of all grades of experience. It has been reported that unlike argon laser trabeculoplasty (Khan et al 1986) the success of trabeculectomy does not depend on the experience of the surgeon (Murray & Jay 1979, Morrell et al 1989).

The lower intraocular pressure and improved visual field survival with early surgery have been described above. Eyes which in retrospect remained controlled on medical therapy without operation showed visual field stability equivalent to those which had early operation. The worst performance, however, was seen in the 55% of eyes in which the initial attempts at medical control proved unsuccessful (Fig. 5.2). An unexpected anomaly was found when eyes with the mildest field loss at diagnosis were compared with those with more severe disease. Over the mean 4.7 years of follow-up, there was little change in visual field in the severe cases whether initially treated conventionally or by early surgery. Similarly, the mild cases treated by early surgery showed little visual field deterioration. The striking deterioration occurred in the eyes with mild field loss at diagnosis during unsuccessful attempts at medical control. This was attributed to the prolonged delay before abandoning medical therapy in these cases. Thus, for cases with mild field

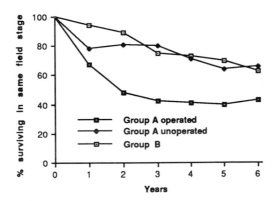

Fig. 5.2 Visual field survival curves showing percentage of eyes remaining in the same stage of the classification for group A (conventional treatment) controlled without operation, group A not controlled without operation and group B (early trabeculectomy). The worst performance is in eyes in which the attempted medical control fails. The eyes which in retrospect could be controlled medically did no better than those treated by early trabeculectomy. (Reproduced with permission from Jay & Allen 1989.)

loss at diagnosis, the mean time of medical therapy before trabeculectomy was 22.9 months, whereas for severe cases it was only 11.4 months. The surgeons' perception of lower risk in the milder cases led to a more prolonged attempt at medical control which proved detrimental. The commonest indication for abandoning medical therapy in the early months was failure to control the intraocular pressure. Later, visual field deterioration with or without an apparently satisfactory intraocular pressure became a more frequent indication. Approximately 70% of the severe cases had required surgery in the first three years compared with 30% of the mild cases. After three years, very few eyes required operation (Fig. 5.3).

The policy of early surgery was also examined for disadvantages. Both groups showed gradual deterioration of visual acuity but there was no significant difference between the groups, although the trend was for slightly more loss of acuity in the conventionally treated group. About 10% of eyes developed lens opacity which reduced the acuity by more than one line of the Snellen chart. This rarely occurred in the 20% of eyes which had mild cataract at the time of diagnosis. The incidence of progressive lens opacity was the same in each group. Perhaps this suggests that it is not only surgical treatment which is responsible for the increased frequency of cataract in glaucoma (Harding & van Heyningen 1987). In the whole conventional treatment group, which required operations in about 50% of cases, the cataract rate was the same as in the early surgery group, 100% of which had operation. Is medical therapy therefore equally cataractogenic? Is delayed surgery more likely to produce cataract or is the risk of cataract merely related to the disease rather than its treatment?

Sudden loss of the last central island of visual field after operation did not occur in this trial. It has been described (Lichter & Ravin 1974) but has not been experienced by all authors (Honrubia et al 1980) and others describe it

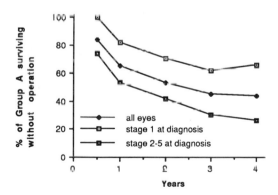

Fig. 5.3 Survival curves for percentage of eyes treated conventionally which remain controlled without operation at each year. Separate curves for whole group data and subgroups according to severity of field loss at diagnosis. Stage 1 eyes have mild relative scotomas. Stages 2–5 have increasing areas of absolute scotomas. The operation rate slows after the first year. (Reproduced with permission from Jay & Allen 1989.)

as a rare event (Aggarwal & Hendeles 1986). Kolker (1986) found its incidence to be similar to that occurring in medically treated cases with equivalent severity of field loss. It should therefore not be used as an excuse to avoid surgery. However, in eyes with only a small terminal island of central field, the risk of early postoperative rise in intraocular pressure should be reduced by giving carbonic anhydrase inhibitors or beta-blocker eye drops at the end of the operation.

As with any form of surgery, there may be complications following glaucoma operations, and a comprehensive review is given by Le Blanc & Stewart (1986). However, serious complications after trabeculectomy seem very rare (Watson et al 1990). If a trial of medical therapy merely delays surgery in many cases, then surgical complications are not avoided. The risk of field loss during attempted medical control outweighs the low risk of serious surgical complications in those eyes which otherwise might be controlled without operation.

The financial cost of a strategy of early trabeculectomy is not greater than conventional management (Ainsworth & Jay 1990). More frequent outpatient visits and higher drug costs for conventional management balanced the cost of extra operations in the early surgery plan. This balance of costs was for an average hospital admission of seven days for each trabeculectomy. If patients are admitted to hospital for a shorter period (current practice varies between one and four days) then the early surgery policy is less expensive. Even at current levels of activity for glaucoma treatment, we can expect an increase in the cost of providing the required care as the average age of the population increases. For Finland, Raivio (1987) has predicted an increased requirement of 40% by the year 2010.

KEY POINTS TO CLINICAL PRACTICE: CHOICE OF TREATMENT FOR DIFFERENT STAGES OF DISEASE

Opinion on the relative merits of medical and surgical treatment have always varied. Ideally, present shift in opinion should be based on more objective research data. In some countries and in some social circumstances, supply or supervision of medical treatment is impracticable and therefore there may be bias in favour of surgical treatment. Where there are optimum conditions for application of all types of therapy, a careful choice should be made depending on the severity of disease. This will be modified where there are doubts about compliance or follow-up, and the patients' own fears, prejudices and life expectancy should be considered. Patients with primary open angle glaucoma seem to have a normal life expectancy for their age (Jay & Murray 1988).

Ocular hypertension without visual field loss

In mild ocular hypertension, for example with pressure less than 30 mmHg and no risk factors for accelerated field loss, observation without treatment is usual. If the pressure is higher than 30 mmHg in the absence of other risk factors, or lower than this in association with risk factors such as family history of glaucoma, optic disc cupping, glaucoma in the fellow eye, diabetes, arterial hypertension, myopia, pseudoexfoliation, aphakia, etc., treatment is required. There is limited information about the relative importance of these various risk factors. Level of intraocular pressure seems most important and David et al (1977) found that a pressure of over 30 mmHg conferred a risk of field loss more than three times that of a pressure between 26 and 30 mmHg. Individually, the other risk factors do not have good predictive value for progressive disease.

When treatment rather than observation is required, the choice is between medical therapy and argon laser trabeculoplasty. Apart from convenience or compliance, there is little practical difference in their effectiveness.

Few surgeons would advocate trabeculectomy when there is no field loss but if the intraocular pressure continues above 30 mmHg, even after other forms of therapy, trabeculectomy may be considered. Most would monitor these cases for deterioration in visual field or optic disc before operating but this plan ignores the possibility of sudden loss of vision caused by retinal vein occlusion.

Established glaucoma with visual field loss

How do recent trials help us to decide on indications and timing of trabeculectomy so that we may avoid detrimental delay, yet prevent unnecessary surgery? If there is a 70% chance of medical therapy being abandoned within three years and if during this period there is field loss which would otherwise be avoided, it is wise to offer trabeculectomy at diagnosis. This is the case where the intraocular pressure is over 30 mmHg before treatment and there are areas of absolute field loss, even if only small in area.

In milder cases, for example, with pressure below 30 mmHg and only relative scotomas, only 30% required operation within three years, but the unsuccessful trial of medical therapy was particularly damaging. It is therefore our current practice to attempt medical or laser control in these milder cases but proceed rapidly to trabeculectomy if the intraocular pressure is not well within the normal range in a few weeks. If the pressure appears satisfactory, close monitoring of visual field should identify those who still deteriorate and trabeculectomy is offered without attempting to restore medical control.

REFERENCES

Aggarwal S P, Hendeles S 1986 Risk of sudden visual loss following trabeculectomy in advanced primary open angle glaucoma. Br J Ophthalmol 70: 97–99
Ainsworth J, Jay J L 1991 Cost analysis of conventional management and early trabeculectomy in the treatment of primary open angle glaucoma. Eye (in press)
Becker B, Morton W R 1966 Topical epinephrine in glaucoma suspects. Am J Ophthalmol 62: 272–277

Boyd T A S 1955 A comparison of surgical and conservative treatments in glaucoma simplex. Trans Ophthalmol Soc UK 75: 541–554

Brown S V L, Thomas J V, Simmons R J 1985 Laser trabeculoplasty re-treatment. Am J Ophthalmol 99: 8–10

Cairns J E 1968 Trabeculectomy: preliminary report of a new method. Am J Ophthalmol 66: 673–679

Cartwright M J, Anderson D R 1988 Correlation of asymmetric damage with asymmetric intraocular pressure in normal tension glaucoma. Arch Ophthalmol 106: 898–900

Chauhan B C, Drance S M, Douglas G R 1989 The time course of intraocular pressure in timolol treated and untreated glaucoma suspects. Am J Ophthalmol 107: 471–475

Committee on Safety of Medicine 1990 Personal communication

Crichton A, Drance S M, Douglas G R et al 1989 Unequal intraocular pressure and its relation to asymmetric visual field defects in low tension glaucoma. Ophthalmology 96: 1312–1314

Crick R P, Vogel R, Newson R B et al 1989 The visual field in chronic simple glaucoma and ocular hypertension: its character, progress, relationship to the level of intraocular pressure and responses to treatment. Eye 3: 536–546

David R, Livingstone D G, Luntz M H 1977 Ocular hypertension: a long term follow up study of treated and untreated patients. Br J Ophthalmol 61: 668–674

de Jong N, Greve E L, Hoynig P F J et al 1989 Results of a filtering procedure in low tension glaucoma. Int Ophthalmol 13: 131–138

Duzanec Z, Krieglstein G K 1981 Correlation between regulation of intraocular pressure, anatomical localisation of trephination and trephine diameter in goniotrephination procedures: a prospective study. Klin Monatsbl Augenheilkd 178: 431–435

Epstein D L, Krug J H, Hertzmark E et al 1989 Long term clinical trial of timolol therapy versus no treatment in management of glaucoma suspects. Ophthalmology 96: 1460–1467

Fink A I, Jordan A J, Lao P N et al 1988 Therapeutic limitation of argon laser trabeculoplasty. Br J Ophthalmol 72: 263–269

Freyler H, Menapace R 1988 Is it possible to avoid blindness due to glaucoma? (Analysis of 121 glaucoma-affected eyes that turned blind despite treatment.) Spektrum Augenheilkd 2: 121–127

Fronimopoulos J, Lambrou N, Pelekis N, Christakis C 1970 Elliotsche Trepanation mit Skleraldekel, Klin Monatsbl Augenheilkd 156: 1–8

Gilbert C M, Brown R H, Lynch M G 1986 The effect of argon laser trabeculoplasty on the rate of filtering surgery. Ophthalmology 93: 362–365

Harding J J, van Heyningen R 1987 Epidemiology and risk factors for cataract. Eye 1: 537–541

Holmin C, Thorburn W, Krakau C E T 1988 Treatment versus no treatment in chronic open angle glaucoma. Acta Ophthalmol 66: 170–173

Honrubia F M, Abad M P, Gomez M L et al 1980 Surgery for pre-terminal glaucoma with residual central 'islet'. Arch Soc Esp Ophthalmol 40: 1228–1232

Hoskins H F Jr, Hetherington J Jr, Minkler D S et al 1983 Complications of laser trabeculoplasty. Ophthalmology 90: 796–799

Jay J L 1983 Earlier trabeculectomy. Trans Ophthalmol Soc UK 103: 35–38

Jay J L, Allen D 1989 The benefit of early trabeculectomy versus conventional management in primary open angle glaucoma relative to severity of disease. Eye 3: 528–535

Jay J L, Murray S B 1980 Characteristics of reduction of intraocular pressure after trabeculectomy. Br J Ophthalmol 100: 432–435

Jay J L, Murray S B 1988 Early trabeculectomy versus conventional management in primary open angle glaucoma. Br J Ophthalmol 72: 881–889

Kass M A, Gordon M, Meltzer D W 1986a Can ophthalmologists correctly identify patients defaulting from pilocarpine therapy? Am J Ophthalmol 101: 524–530

Kass M A, Meltzer D W, Gordon I M et al 1986b Compliance with topical pilocarpine treatment. Am J Ophthalmol 101: 515–523

Kass M A, Gordon M, Morley R E et al 1987 Compliance with topical timolol treatment. Am J Ophthalmol 103: 188–193

Khan K A, Lederer C M Jr, Willoughby L 1986 Argon laser trabeculoplasty in a residency program. Ophthalmic Surg 17: 343–350

Kidd M N, O'Connor M 1985 Progression of field loss after trabeculectomy: a five-year follow-up. Br J Ophthalmol 69: 827–831

Kolker A E 1986 Visual prognosis in advanced glaucoma. In: Cairns J (ed) Glaucoma. Grune & Stratton, London, pp 647–660

Le Blanc R P, Stewart R H 1986 Complications of glaucoma surgery. In: Weinstein G W (ed) Open angle glaucoma. Churchill Livingstone, Edinburgh, pp 183–200

Lehmann F A, Faggioni R 1986 Two years experience with argon laser trabeculoplasty. Klin Monatsbl Augenheilkd 188: 519–522

Lichter P R, Ravin J G 1974 Risks of sudden visual loss after glaucoma surgery. Am J Ophthalmol 78: 1009–1013

Lund O E, Zink H 1988 Long term results of argon laser trabeculoplasty. Klin Monatsbl Augenheilkd 193: 572–578

Migdal C, Hitchings R 1986 Control of chronic simple glaucoma with primary medical, surgical and laser treatment. Trans Ophthalmol Soc UK 105: 653–656

Miller K M, Quigley H A 1988 The clinical appearance of the lamina cribrosa as a function of the extent of glaucomatous optic nerve damage. Ophthalmology 95: 135–138

Morrell A J, Searle A E T, O'Neil E C 1989 Trabeculectomy as an introduction to intraocular surgery in an ophthalmic training program. Ophthalmic Surg 20: 557–560

Moulin F, Haut J, Abi Rached J 1987 Late failures of trabeculoplasty. Int Ophthalmol 10: 61–66

Murray S B, Jay J L 1979 Trabeculectomy: its role in the management of glaucoma. Trans Ophthalmol Soc UK 99: 492–494

Odberg T 1987 Visual field prognosis in advanced glaucoma. Acta Ophthalmol 65 (suppl 182): 27–29

Osusky R 1986 Long term observation of goniotrephination with different trephine diameters. Klin Monatsbl Augenheilkd 189: 398–399

Parrish R K, Folberg R 1989 Wound healing in glaucoma surgery. In: Ritch R, Shields M B, Krupin T (eds) The glaucomas. Mosby, St Louis, pp 633–643

Parsley J, Powell R G, Keightley S J et al 1987 Postural response of intraocular pressure in chronic open angle glaucoma following trabeculectomy. Br J Ophthalmol 77: 494–496

Raivio I 1987 Number of glaucoma patients in Finland in the year 2010. Acta Ophthalmol 65 (suppl 182): 21–23

Richter C U, Shingleton B J, Bellows A R et al 1987 Retreatment with argon laser trabeculoplasty. Ophthalmology 94: 1085–1089

Richter C U, Shingleton B J, Bellows A R et al 1988 The development of encapsulated filtering blebs. Ophthalmology 95: 1163–1168

Rouhiainen H, Terasvirta M 1988 Repeated 50 burn 1180 degree argon laser trabeculoplasty. Acta Opthalmol 66: 83–86

Schwartz A L, Love D C, Schwartz M A 1985 Long term follow up of argon laser trabeculoplasty for uncontrolled open angle glaucoma. Arch Ophthalmol 103: 1482–1484

Scott D R, Quigley H A 1988 Medical management of a high bleb phase after trabeculectomies. Ophthalmology 95: 1169–1173

Sherwood M B, Grierson I, Miller L et al 1989 Long term morphologic effects of anti glaucoma drugs on the conjunctiva and Tenon's capsule in glaucomatous patients. Ophthalmology 96: 327–335

Shingleton B J, Richter C U, Bellows A R et al 1990 Management of encapsulated filtration blebs. Ophthalmology 97: 63–68

Smith R J H 1972 Medical versus surgical therapy in glaucoma simplex. Br J Ophthalmol 56: 277–283

Smith R J H 1986 The enigma of primary open angle glaucoma. Trans Ophthalmol Soc UK

105: 618–633

Sponsel W E 1989 Tonometry in question: can visual screening tests play a more decisive role in glaucoma diagnosis and management? Surv Ophthalmol 33 (suppl): 291–300

Starita R J, Fellman R L, Spaeth G L et al 1985 Short and long term effects of post-operative corticosteroids on trabeculectomy. Ophthalmology 92: 938–945

Tauber J, Melamed S, Foster C D 1989 Glaucoma in patients with ocular cicatricial pemphigoid. Ophthalmology 96: 33–37

Thomas R, Jay L 1988 Raised intraocular pressure with topical steroids after trabeculectomy. Graefe's Arch Clin Exp Ophthalmol 226: 337–340

Ticho U, Nescher R 1989 Laser trabeculoplasty in glaucoma: ten year evaluation. Arch Ophthalmol 107: 844–846

Tuulonen A, Niva A K, Alanko H I 1987 A controlled five-year follow-up study of laser trabeculoplasty as primary therapy for open angle glaucoma. Am J Ophthalmol 104: 334–338

Tuulonen A, Koponen J, Alanko H I et al 1989 Laser trabeculoplasty versus medication treatment as primary therapy for glaucoma. Acta Ophthalmol 67: 275–280

Watson P G 1970 Trabeculectomy: a modified ab externo technique. Ann Ophthalmol 2: 199–205

Watson P G, Jakeman M, Ozturk M F et al 1990 The complications of trabeculectomy (A 20 year follow-up). Eye 4: 425–438

Werner E B, Drance S M, Schulzer M 1977 Trabeculectomy and the progression of glaucomatous visual field loss. Arch Ophthalmol 95: 1374–1377

Wilke K, Storr–Paulsen A 1986 Indications of trabeculectomy in open angle glaucoma. Acta Ophthalmol 64: 258–262

Wise J B 1987 10 year results of laser trabeculoplasty. Eye 1: 45–50

Wise J B, Witter 1979 Argon laser therapy for open angle glaucoma: a pilot study. Arch Ophthalmol 97: 319–322

6

Automated perimetry

P. K. Wishart

INTRODUCTION

Automated perimetry (AP) has been described as the best diagnostic method the ophthalmologist has for both the detection and the routine clinical management of open angle glaucoma (OAG) (Lewis & Johnson 1985, Heuer 1988, Greve et al 1985). Many clinicians, however, are unaware of the advantages of AP and the help it offers in facing the major challenge of the diagnosis of early glaucoma. This chapter is intended to give the clinician who is unfamiliar with AP an introduction to the subject and its clinical usefulness, as well as to dispel some of the arguments against its use. These arguments include the beliefs that automated perimetry is too time consuming to be practical, too complicated to allow patient cooperation, and presents too much detailed and confusing information to be helpful.

In the knowledge that the majority of patients with ocular hypertension do not progress to OAG (Perkins 1973, Wilensky et al 1974, Kitazawa et al 1977), the ophthalmologist cannot give treatment on the basis of raised intraocular pressure (IOP) alone. However, indecision and doubt affect our judgment because of our relative inadequacy in diagnosing and detecting the condition in its earliest stages, especially as recent studies have documented that significant glaucomatous damage may have occurred prior to visible nerve fibre layer (NFL) loss (Quigley & Addicks 1982, Katsumori & Mizokami 1989) or abnormalities of perimetry (Quigley et al 1982).

The problem in diagnosing OAG is that the clinician must employ a test that is suitably sensitive to detect early glaucoma but specific enough not to falsely identify normals as glaucomatous. The test must also be within the capacity of the patient's cooperation and quick enough to be widely available. Automated perimetry goes a long way to meeting most of these stipulations, and as well as offering the clinician his most useful means of help in the management of glaucoma, automated perimetry is allowing major advances into research and contributing greatly to our understanding of glaucoma.

EARLY STRUCTURAL AND FUNCTIONAL CHANGES IN OAG

If we examine the ideal conditions for and characteristics of a suitable test for the diagnosis and clinical management of glaucoma, at present only visual field analysis offers a scientific and quantifiable method. The range of IOP in normal eyes is so wide that it is not a quantifiable management parameter in OAG. Optic disc examination often allows prediction of visual field defects by an experienced observer, but there are limitations to the information that can be gained from examining the optic disc (Drance 1978, Hitchings & Spaeth 1977). Monocular examination of the optic disc is adequate only in the detection of some specific features indicative of glaucomatous damage such as the presence of rim haemorrhages, notching of the neural rim or bayonetting of vessels at the disc edge. Saucerization of the nerve head is an important feature of glaucomatous damage yet this is only visible on stereoscopic examination. The time-honoured cup disc ratio is now understood to represent nothing more than the relative size of the optic canal through which the optic nerve head passes (Quigley 1985). It is the neuroretinal rim area that is important and not the cup size per se (Airaksinen et al 1985). The increased resolution provided by the slit-lamp biomicroscope is necessary for accurate assessment of the optic disc (Hoskins & Gelber 1975). Tuulonen et al (1987) have shown the importance of optic disc pallor in glaucomatous change in the optic disc, and defects in the NFL of the retina are known to be one of the earliest features of glaucomatous damage (Airaksinen et al 1984), but these defects may be very difficult to detect unless sophisticated photographic techniques are used. Stereophotography of the optic disc is superior to fundus drawing for recognizing glaucomatous damage (Sommer et al 1979), but miosis and lens opacity may prevent some features of disc damage being adequately represented, and, as with NFL photography, does not represent a useful means of monitoring the patient's progress.

There have been strenuous attempts to develop a truly objective test which would show early glaucomatous optic nerve damage not dependent on the patient's cooperation, and reproducible in all circumstances. Psychophysical tests of optic nerve function such as contrast sensitivity (Arden & Jacobson 1978), colour vision, peripheral displacement thresholds (Fitzke et al 1989), pattern electroretinography (Wanger & Persson 1987), flash and flicker visual evoked potentials (Schmeisser & Smith 1989) have all been shown recently to yield evidence of abnormality in glaucomatous subjects. However, as yet no test has been discovered that will effectively remove all uncertainty in the diagnosis of glaucoma. Essentially psychophysical tests are relatively unquantifiable and many of these tests may still be affected by the patient's subjectivity and by factors such as degree of lens opacity, patient's age and learning effects (Drance et al 1989). The results of psychophysical tests in normal eyes cover such a wide range that it may be difficult to differentiate a pathological result from a normal result. Quigley (1989) has suggested that the decrease of function with age in psychophysical testing may represent degenerative age changes at the retinal photoreceptor level rather than decreased function of the ganglion cell layer and optic nerve.

Hopefully, further research will provide improved methods of diagnosis and measurement of glaucomatous damage but at the moment, as has been the case for many years, visual field analysis remains the best and most routinely available method.

VISUAL FIELD ANALYSIS IN THE DIAGNOSIS AND MANAGEMENT OF OAG

Having decided therefore that visual field analysis is the way we wish to diagnose and monitor our glaucoma patients we must examine the techniques available for this purpose. Some clinicians today feel that a search for simplicity justifies adherence to older and simpler methods rather than automated perimetry. When presented with an automated perimeter capable of conducting a whole range of visual field tests the ophthalmologist may be bewildered by the apparent complexities of the test and of the technical language used to explain these tests.

Alternative methods of perimetry

Goldmann perimetry, until the advent of automated perimetry, was the standard method of field analysis in the USA. Few centres in the UK possess the highly trained technician necessary to produce good Goldmann fields, and simpler methods have been relied on. An idea of the training required by a Goldmann perimetrist was emphasized recently by Dunbar Hoskins (1989), who reported he had undergone three months' training during a glaucoma fellowship before he felt fully competent to chart accurately glaucomatous visual field loss with the Goldmann perimeter. Three minutes' experience with Goldmann perimetry may be all that most ophthalmologists in training in the UK receive. It is perhaps a consequence of their relative unfamiliarity with Goldmann perimetry that makes understanding of automated perimetry, which is based on the Goldmann, seem difficult to some UK clinicians.

Automated perimetry offers major advantages over manual perimetry that readily become apparent to the clinician when this newer method of field analysis is employed. First, it is necessary to consider the reasons for the international acceptance that Goldmann perimetry achieved prior to the advent of AP. Goldmann perimetry allows accurate, precise and quantifiable documentation of a patient's field of vision and demonstration of the size and depths of any scotomas identified. Goldmann perimetry, which may be performed with both kinetic and static presentation of stimuli, offered new standards of precision and quantification of visual field loss compared to other manual methods such as the tangent screen and Lister perimeter. The major disadvantage of manual field analysis with methods other than Goldmann (and confrontation) is that fixation cannot be monitored, and quantification of field loss is relatively imprecise. The major disadvantages to Goldmann perimetry are that it requires a highly trained perimetrist, it is time consuming and prone to procedure-induced error.

In the detection of glaucomatous defects, static perimetry with the Tubingen perimeter has been shown to be superior to Goldmann kinetic perimetry (Portney & Krohn 1978, Aulhorn & Harms 1967). Similarly, automated perimetry has been shown to be superior to manual static perimetry in detecting early glaucomatous visual field defects (Heijl 1976). Beck et al (1985) showed that automated perimetry detected field loss in 21% of suspects classed as normal with manual techniques, while Azuma & Tokuoka (1987) found field loss with automated perimetry in 16% of eyes classed as normal after manual perimetry. Quigley et al (1982) has shown that up to 40% of nerve fibres may be lost despite normal Goldmann perimetry. With automated perimetry, he has shown that earlier detection of field loss is possible, and if damage is localized visual field loss may be detected when only 5% of ganglion cells have been lost (Quigley et al 1989).

Static perimetry using semi-automatic perimeters such as the Friedmann field analyser utilizes suprathreshold testing at specific points in the central 25° of the field. Only a relatively crude estimate of the patient's hill of vision is obtainable with this method of perimetry, although its sensitivity in detecting early field loss in one study was reported to be as good as that of the Goldmann perimeter (Batko et al 1983). However, suprathreshold testing is not regarded as an adequate method of monitoring the progression of glaucomatous field loss (Gloor et al 1987, Batko et al 1983), as progression may be by deepening of existing defects (Mikelberg & Drance 1984). The more accurate and more sensitive field analysis with automated perimetry will show pathology earlier than cruder non-automated methods and allow accurate quantification of this damage.

Benefits of automated perimetry

The advantages of automation over Goldmann perimetry fall into four major categories:

1. Standardization of the testing procedure
2. Improved sensitivity, accuracy, quantification and repeatability in the detection of field loss
3. Objective assessment of the patient's performance
4. Easy interpretation and statistical analysis of test results.

With AP, a trained perimetrist is not required as the technical expertise to perform perimetry is contained within the computer software. With the Goldmann perimeter, accurate calibration of both stimulus and background illumination must be performed daily to ensure repeatable results. AP overcomes these possible errors in testing procedure, by eliminating the perimetrist and ensuring self-calibration.

Automated perimetry improves accuracy of detection of visual field loss by performing static threshold estimations of retinal sensitivity with randomized stimulus presentation and optimal stimulus duration. The computer programs which govern the testing procedure give rise to the third major category of advantages — assessment of the reliability of the patient by monitoring the patient's performance throughout the test. Most patients are motivated by the desire to see as many stimuli as possible and will therefore consciously or unconsciously tend to lose fixation and seek stimuli where they expect them. With AP, fixation is monitored independently of the technician by occasionally presenting a stimulus in the predetermined area of the patient's blind spot. If the patient responds to this stimulus, then his fixation must have wandered. In addition, a video monitor allows the technician to ensure that the eye is centrally placed behind the trial lens and that this position is maintained throughout the test. To detect the 'trigger-happy' patient (false positives) the machine occasionally makes the noise associated with stimulus presentation at a time when no stimulus is presented. A high false-positive score detected by this method invalidates the result. Similarly, the inattentive patient is recognized when a stimulus in an area of the visual field he has previously responded to is not identified on repeat presentation (false-negative score). Thus AP is the only technique available for monitoring the visual fields in which the clinician has a very accurate estimation of how well the patient coped with the test. Obviously, an apparent change in the visual field should not lead to a change in treatment if the field analysis is shown to be unreliable.

The argument suggested by some clinicians that a high degree of sophistication in the patient must be necessary to cooperate with computerized perimetry has been disproved by Traverso et al (1987), who demonstrated that in a population of illiterate rural patients in Saudi Arabia with no previous experience of perimetry accurate results were achieved with automated visual field analysis.

Keltner & Johnson (1983) have shown that it is possible to obtain as much or more visual information with AP in 10 minutes than can be obtained in 1 hour of manual testing. A screening programme on the Humphrey Field Analyser will take approximately 5–7 minutes per eye and is quicker and more sensitive than manual screening methods (Kosoko et al 1986, Mundorf et al 1989).

AP affords random presentation of stimuli over the area of the field tested, which overcomes the patient's tendency to predict the appearance of the next stimulus. Further standardization is achieved by fixing the duration of the stimulus presentation to 0.2 seconds, which is regarded as optimal for physiological summation of retinal stimuli to occur without permitting involuntary eye movements (Perimetric Standards 1979).

TECHNICAL ASPECTS OF PROJECTION PERIMETRY

The basic principle of perimetry is to obtain a measurement of the eye's indirect vision by determining the peripheral limits of vision, and the retinal sensitivity (its ability to discriminate different light intensities) within those limits. This is essentially a mapping of the 'hill of vision'. The lowest level of illumination that can be perceived at the retina is termed the retinal threshold for that point. Below this threshold, a stimulus is too dim to be perceived, and the more intense (the brighter the stimulus) than threshold the easier such a stimulus should be seen. Such a stimulus is termed suprathreshold. As there is a zone around the threshold point in which stimuli may sometimes be seen and sometimes not, suprathreshold testing is a method used in screening techniques to limit the number of false-positive responses, i.e. where a point of normal retinal sensitivity failed to detect a stimulus not quite bright enough at that point in time to be perceived. The higher the retinal threshold the more sensitive are the retinal receptors at that point and the dimmer the stimuli which may be perceived. Some confusion often arises over the nomenclature used to record the various optical parameters used in different perimeters.

The ratio of two powers in a mechanical system is expressed in logarithmic units called decibels. The intensity of light is measured in apostilbs (Asb). However, as visual perception seems to relate to ratios between light intensities rather than to the difference between them, the attenuation of light is measured in logarithmic units – decibels (Anderson 1987). Thus retinal sensitivity is expressed in decibels. The light of a projected spot in a bowl perimeter is attenuated by neutral density filters measured in log units (decibels), with 1 log unit equal to 10 decibels (dB). If a point on the retina can be found to respond to light of intensity reduced to one-tenth of its value by a 1 log unit filter (10 dB) and no dimmer, then the retinal threshold of that point is 10 dB. A 2 log unit (20-dB) filter reduces the light intensity to one-hundredth of its original value. If this light is perceived, the retinal sensitivity is 20 dB, and if light is still perceived when a 3 log unit filter (30 dB) reduces the light to one-thousandth of its intensity, the retinal sensitivity will be 30 dB. Thus the greater the attenuation of light, the dimmer the stimulus and, if perceived, the higher the retinal threshold (sensitivity).

In Goldmann perimetry the graded spot sizes and attenuating filters allow stimuli to be presented over the range of 1–1000 asb in grades of 0.1 log unit. All points corresponding to one level of intensity are joined by a line called an isopter. As retinal sensitivity increases towards the fovea successively smaller or dimmer spot sizes can be perceived. As well as being used for kinetic perimetry the Goldmann perimeter can take static cuts by determining the retinal threshold along a preselected meridian.

Static perimetry with the Goldmann perimeter is a laborious task and is only usually performed along meridians in which there is an expected defect. AP, however, performs static threshold testing in which the retinal sensitivity is tested at multiple points in the visual field, the location of the points depending on the particular programme selected. The brightness of the projected spot in automated bowl perimeters such as the Octopus or the Humphrey Field Analyser is decreased by successive attenuation of filters in 4-dB steps (0.4 of a log unit) until the stimulus is too dim to be perceived. The illumination of the spot is then increased in 2-dB steps until the patient responds to the stimulus. The illumination is then decreased and successively increased to 'fine tune' the stimulus and obtain a precise threshold measurement. This target bracketing – the 'staircase' technique of threshold determination – allows an exceptionally precise and accurate determination of the retinal threshold of seeing over each tested point on the hill of vision. In general the distance between tested points in AP is 6° and this has been shown to maintain the best balance between the sensitivity of the test (i.e. significant scotomas are unlikely not to impinge on a grid of points with this separation) and the time necessary to conduct the test.

Interpreting the results of automated perimetry

The interpretation of results provided by some of the earlier automated perimeters was very difficult because of the wealth of numerical data supplied, and considerable time and energy were necessary to gain any useful appreciation of the results of the test. Modern perimeters like the newer generation of the Octopus perimeters and the Humphrey Field Analyser, especially when used with the Statpac program (Statistical Analysis Package), resolve these problems entirely as the computer software analyses the raw data and presents it in a readily understandable form. A grey scale shows a map of the hill of vision, with darkness proportional to loss of sensitivity. The difference from the expected result in the visual field is displayed numerically, as is the difference from the normal age-matched population. Finally a probability chart shows for each defect the likelihood of this being a variation of normal.

Visual field indices

Interpretation and comparison of serial visual fields with AP is facilitated by measurements called visual field indices or global indices (Flammer et al 1985). These indices are the mean deviation (MD), the short-term fluctuation (SF) and the corrected loss variance (CLV). The mean deviation (or deficit) in decibels – either elevation or depression – from a normal age-matched population is presented showing overall difference in sensitivity from normal. A depression of this value is indicative of glaucoma in the absence of other pathology. The short-term fluctuation is recorded by retesting points throughout the test, and is a measurement by which the threshold fluctuates between seeing and not seeing during the course of the test. A high short-term fluctuation appearing on a field whose reliability parameters are good may be one of the first signs of glaucomatous damage (Flammer et al 1984). The computer then calculates the CLV. This value is calculated from the difference between the test results and the expected results from an age-matched normal database with the short-term fluctuation taken into account. A localized scotoma will cause little depression of the MD, but will give rise to an abnormal CLV as this measurement corrects for intratest variability. Thus instead of concerning himself with a bewildering array of threshold values the clinician looks at the grey scale to gain an overall impression of the health of the visual field, then reads the values for the MD, SF and CLV which have been shown to be highly sensitive indicators of glaucomatous damage and allow for easy comparison with future field tests (Flammer & Drance 1985).

Serial field analysis with automated perimetry

Another problem with manual and semi-automated perimetry is the comparison of serial fields. It is very difficult to compare one field to the next and say whether there has been an overall progression of field loss, especially if there is a relative improvement in one part of the field and a worsening in another. This problem is also solved for the clinician who uses AP with a statistical analysis program such as the Humphrey Statpac. Here the physician can ask the computer to present an analysis of all previously stored visual fields on a patient's eye. An easily understandable graphic display is produced, showing the spread of the threshold measurements represented as a box plot indicating mean deviation from normal and displaying the peaks and troughs of sensitivity with the spread and position of the 'box' proportional to the net increase or decrease of sensitivity of the field. If five or more fields of similar strategy have been performed, the computer performs a linear regression analysis of the slope of the mean deviation, informing the examiner whether there has been a statistically significant change in the patient's field.

AUTOMATED PERIMETRY IN CLINICAL PRACTICE

Two examples are given to show the usefulness of appropriate automated perimetry. The right optic discs of each of the two patients are shown in Figures 6.1 and 6.2. In case A, a large vertically oval cup is seen with pathological notching of the superior rim. In case B marked pallor and thinning of the neuro-retinal rim indicative of advanced glaucoma is seen. Both were relatively young patients presenting in one case (case A) with borderline elevation of IOP, and in the other (case B) with normal IOP, but with a history of isolated episodes of IOP elevation detected by his optician. The grey-scale print-out of both cases is shown in Figures 6.3 and 6.4. The box-plot serial comparison of the patients' fields are shown in Figures 6.5 (case A) and 6.6 (case B). The dense inferior arcuate scotoma in case A is shown not to worsen in the subsequent box-plot representations of the field tests. Linear regression analysis performed by the Field Analyser shows that there is no significant change in the slope of MD in this series of fields compared to normal. In case B, however, after an initial test which showed marked field loss and high short-term fluctuation and poor reliability parameters, the subsequent field improved. Thereafter, his field loss worsened as shown by a significant worsening of the slope of mean deviation from normal by linear regression analysis.

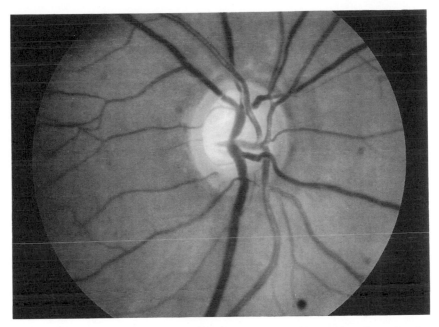

Fig. 6.1 Case A: right optic disc   increased vertical cupping with notching of superior rim.

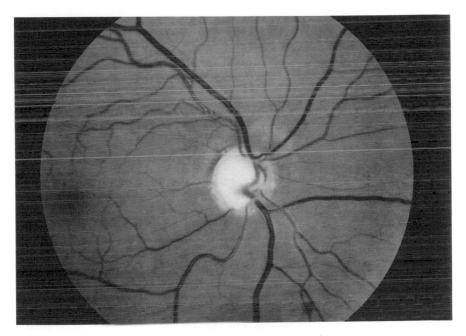

Fig. 6.2 Case B: right optic disc – advanced glaucomatous cupping.

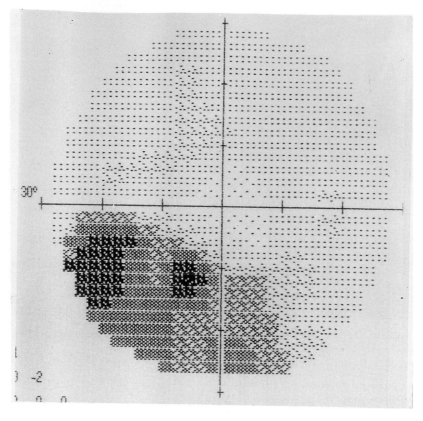

Fig. 6.3   Grey-scale representation of visual field in case A, showing inferior arcuate scotoma with nasal step.

All properly conducted visual field testing, including AP, is relatively time consuming, but the time spent on AP because of its standardization, its sensitivity, its reproducibility and its reliability, may represent a much better investment of time than that spent in performing relatively unquantifiable manual perimetry. Careful clinical selection is necessary to optimize the use of this valuable instrument. It may be argued that in most cases of far-advanced glaucoma the patients will probably be on maximum medical treatment and decisions are most likely to be based on IOP levels, the tolerance of treatment and the surgical outlook of the ophthalmologist. Therefore further attempted quantification of advanced field loss is pointless, especially as approximately 5000 nerve fibres per year are lost in the normal optic nerve as a result of ageing (Balaszi et al 1984), and in a grossly damaged optic nerve this loss may represent a considerable proportion. A further proportion of patients may have general or ocular conditions such as senility, retinal vein occlusion or significant lens opacity that may make visual field analysis unrewarding (Beck & Karseras 1982). Accurate visual field testing

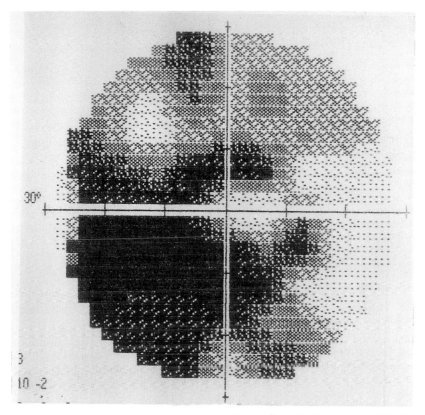

Fig. 6.4 Grey-scale representation of visual field in case B, showing inferior and superior arcuate scotomas encircling fixation with profound loss of inferior nasal aspect of field.

with AP may therefore be used mostly for glaucoma suspects or patients with early glaucoma where the demonstration of visual field loss will be of most importance with regard to the initiation or the change of treatment.

AP has considerably more flexibility than may at first be apparent, and the clinician can reduce the time required for field estimations by varying the strategies available depending on his requirements. It is helpful when performing AP on a patient new to perimetry to use one of the screening strategies as this will be quicker to perform than a full thresholding test and allows the patient to become familiar with the procedure. Screening programmes use suprathreshold testing and will, depending on the strategy, identify a tested point as seen or not seen. The brightness level at which the screening programme is conducted is determined according to the range of normal values expected in that age group. In the case of the Humphrey Field Analyser, the brightness level is determined for the test by first performing a threshold estimation for one point in each of the four quadrants of the field and then suprathreshold testing is conducted relative to this baseline. If a defect is evident and more information is required without thresholding all

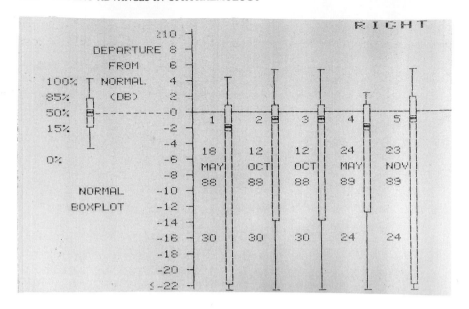

Fig. 6.5 Humphrey 'box-plot' representation of five serial fields in case A. (Three horizontal bars within each box indicating median value show little change.)

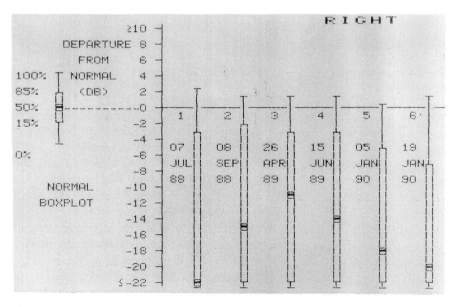

Fig. 6.6 Humphrey 'box-plot' representation of six serial fields in case B. (Three horizontal bars indicating median show significant worsening of median sensitivity from third field on.)

points, then a 'quantify defects' strategy may be used in which the defect depth in decibels is determined for the points not seen with suprathreshold testing.

A full thresholding test may take 10 to 12 minutes to plot the visual field of an eye, but all the information gathered is automatically stored in the computer's memory and can be used to reduce testing time for subsequent tests. Using this previously determined data, threshold testing can start at the expected 'fine tuning' level of 2-dB increments at the previously recorded threshold level. Alternatively a fast thresholding test can be used for follow-up where the entire field is retested at 2-dB brighter than previous values. Any point which is not seen at this new level must have lost sensitivity since the previous test, and such a point will be retested to establish its new threshold. These programmes significantly reduce the time necessary for repeat threshold examinations (to less than 3 minutes with the 'fast threshold') once a satisfactory threshold test is stored in the computer's memory.

Automated perimetry is of course equally sensitive in the detection of neurological field defects as it is at the demonstration of glaucomatous field loss, and again offers the advantages of standardization of testing with high sensitivity, allowing accurate searches for neurological field defects.

GLAUCOMA RESEARCH AND AUTOMATED PERIMETRY

Although this brief summary of the capabilities of AP is largely aimed at the clinician presently undecided as to whether to commit himself to this method of field analysis, the importance of AP to the basic understanding of and research into OAG deserves mentioning. The very sensitivity of AP has greatly increased our knowledge and understanding of the process of glaucomatous visual field loss. Short-term fluctuation in retinal sensitivity was difficult to quantify before the advent of AP, which rapidly and routinely measures it. While a high short-term fluctuation value may be an early indication of glaucomatous damage, it may be due to other factors such as temporary ill health (Langerhorst et al 1989a) and therefore may be responsible for an apparent change in the visual field which might otherwise have been taken to represent progression. Similarly, AP has given unequivocal proof of long-term fluctuation – i.e. a change occurring between two visual fields without a worsening of pathology – and again this has modified our approach to the appraisal of field loss. It is now realized that to document progression of field loss confidently the same trend must be shown in four or preferably five serial fields (Wu et al 1987, Hitchings 1988). Otherwise an apparent change may only represent long-term fluctuation (Wilensky & Joondeph 1984), which AP has shown to increase with age (Katz & Sommer 1987). Once again, such precise information was difficult if not impossible to determine with manual perimetry where, for instance, a differing speed of target presentation might be enough to create an apparent difference between two successive field tests (Johnson & Keltner 1987). It is encouraging to note that a significant learning effect does not occur with AP and therefore any major change occurring between fields after an initial 'baseline' field is likely to be of clinical significance (Werner et al 1988).

Perhaps of greatest importance is the adoption of AP in glaucoma research centres throughout the world (Hoskins 1989). Research workers in different countries can now compare their results with standardized techniques of field analysis without the uncertainties to which different methodology and techniques give rise. The precision offered by AP allows much more accurate judgments of the influence of treatment on the course of the disease to be proven. Using AP Krakau & Holmin (1987) showed progressive field loss to be unaffected by the pressure-lowering effect of argon laser trabeculoplasty in a group of patients with OAG. Such results could easily be open to question if there was the possibility of unreliable or inaccurate field analysis. Other research workers, again using standardized AP to determine results, have confirmed that progression of field loss in OAG can occur despite pressure lowering by argon laser trabeculoplasty (Heijl & Bengtsson 1984, Drance et al 1987). These results cast doubt on one of the fundamental tenets in our management of OAG – that of the field-preserving effect of IOP reduction (Heijl 1989). Furthermore, the world-wide research efforts into developing newer methods of detecting and demonstrating glaucomatous damage all now use AP as a reference standard. Thus with a standardized technique and removal of observer bias and interpretation, one group of research workers comparing a treatment or a test in one centre can tell if their population studied was equivalent to and their results comparable to that of a study elsewhere.

KEY POINTS TO CLINICAL PRACTICE

1.   AP permits high quality and reliable visual field testing free from technician bias and procedure-induced error.

2.   AP allows simple interpretation of sophisticated results.

3.   AP is equally useful for the earliest detection of glaucomatous defects, in screening programmes and for precise quantification and future comparison of documented field loss.

4.   AP identifies unreliable test results and patients whose consistently unreliable responses demonstrate their unsuitability for further perimetry.

5.   Optimal use of AP requires the clinician to exercise judgment in requesting test strategies appropriate to the patient and to the clinician's philosophy of treatment for OAG.

REFERENCES

Airaksinen P J, Drance S M, Douglas G R et al 1984 Diffuse and localized nerve fibre loss in glaucoma. Am J Ophthalmol 98: 566–571
Airaksinen P J, Drance S M, Schulzer M 1985 Neuroretinal rim area in early glaucoma. Am

J Ophthalmol 99: 1–8

Anderson D R 1987 Instruments and strategies. In: Perimetry with and without automation. Mosby, St Louis, pp 32–33

Arden G B, Jacobson J J 1978 A simple grading test for contrast sensitivity: preliminary results indicate value in screening for glaucoma. Invest Ophthalmol Vis Sci 17: 23–27

Aulhorn E, Harms H 1967 Early visual field defects in glaucoma. In: Leydecker W (ed) Glaucoma symposium, Tutzing Castle 1966. Karger, Basel, pp 151–186

Azuma I, Tokuoka S 1987 The usefulness of automated perimetry in detecting early glaucoma. In: Greve E L, Heijl A (eds) 7th International visual fields symposium. Doc Ophthalmol Proc Ser, Nijhoff/Junk, Dordrecht 49: 391–396

Balaszi A G, Rootman J, Drance S M 1984 The effect of age on the nerve fibers population of the human optic nerve. Am J Ophthalmol 97: 760–766

Batko K A, Anctil J L, Anderson D R 1983 Detecting glaucomatous damage with the Friedmann analyser compared with the Goldmann perimeter and evaluation of stereoscopic photographs of the optic disk. Am J Ophthalmol 95: 435–447

Beck M, Karseras A G 1982 Disc assessment and visual field analysis in a hospital glaucoma population. Br J Ophthalmol 66: 99–101

Beck R W, Bergstrom T J, Lichter P R 1985 A clinical comparison of visual field testing with a new automated perimeter, the Humphrey Field Analyzer, and the Goldmann perimeter. Ophthalmology 92: 77–82

Drance S M 1978 The disc and the field in glaucoma. Ophthalmology 85: 209–214

Drance S M, Douglas G R, Schulzer M et al 1987 The effect of laser trabeculoplasty on intraocular pressure and some visual functions. In: Kriegelstein G K (ed) Glaucoma update III. Springer-Verlag, Berlin, pp 207–214

Drance S M, Douglas G R, Schulzer M, Wijsman C S 1989 The learning effect of the Frisen high pass resolution perimeter. In: Heijl A (ed) Perimetry update 1988/89, Proceedings of the VIIIth International Perimetric Society Meeting. Kugler & Ghedini, Amsterdam, pp 199–201

Fitzke F W, Poinoosawmy D, Nagasubramanian S, Hitchings R A 1989 Peripheral displacement thresholds in glaucoma and ocular hypertension. In: Heijl A (ed) Perimetry update 1988/89, Proceedings of the VIIIth International Perimetric Society Meeting. Kugler & Ghedini, Amsterdam, pp 399–405

Flammer J, Drance S M 1985 Quantification of glaucomatous visual field defects with automated perimetry. Chibret Int J Ophthalmol 3: 2–9

Flammer J, Drance S M, Zulauf M 1984 Differential light threshold: short- and long-term fluctuation in patients with glaucoma, normal controls and patients with suspected glaucoma. Arch Ophthalmol 102: 704–706

Flammer J, Drance S M, Augustiny L, Funkhouser A 1985 Quantification of glaucoma visual field defects with automated perimetry. Invest Ophthalmol Vis Sci 26: 176–181

Gloor B, Dimitrakos S A, Rabineau P A 1987 Long-term follow-up of glaucomatous fields by computerized (Octopus) perimetry. In: Kriegelstein G K (ed) Glaucoma update III. Springer Verlag, Berlin, pp 128–138

Greve E L, van den Berg T J T P, Langerhorst C 1985 Present and future of computer assisted perimetry in glaucoma: selected topics. Doc Ophthalmol Proc Ser 43: 1–9

Heijl A 1976 Automatic perimetry in glaucoma visual field screening: a clinical study. Graefes Arch Clin Exp Ophthalmol 200: 21–37

Heijl A 1989 Effect of IOP on the visual field in ocular hypertension and glaucoma. Int Ophthalmol 13: 119–124

Heijl A, Bengtsson B 1984 The effect of laser induced intraocular pressure reduction on the visual field. Acta Ophthalmol 62: 705–714

Heuer D K 1988 Glaucoma update. Ophthalmology 95: 282–287

Hitchings R A 1988 Low tension glaucoma: is treatment worthwhile? Eye 2: 636–640

Hitchings R A, Spaeth G L 1977 The optic disc in glaucoma. II. Correlation of the appearance of the optic disc with the visual field. Br J Ophthalmol 61: 107–113

Hoskins H D 1989 Automated perimetry: presented at the Cambridge symposium on visual field analysis, February 1989

Hoskins H D, Gelber E D 1975 Optic disc topography and visual field defects in patients with increased intraocular pressure. Am J Ophthalmol 80: 284–290

Johnson C A, Keltner J L 1987 Optimal rates of movement for kinetic perimetry. Arch Ophthalmol 105: 73–75

Katsumori N, Mizokami K 1989 Clinicopathological studies of the retinal nerve fibre layer in early glaucomatous visual field damage. In: Heijl A (ed) Perimetry update 1988/89. Kugler & Ghedini, Amsterdam, pp 289–295

Katz J, Sommer A 1987 A longitudinal study of the age-adjusted variability of automated visual fields. Arch Ophthalmol 105: 1083–1086

Kitazawa Y, Horie T, Aoki S et al 1977 Untreated ocular hypertension: a long-term prospective study. Arch Ophthalmol 95: 1180–1184

Keltner J L, Johnson C A 1983 Screening for visual field abnormalities with automated perimetry. Surv Ophthalmol 28: 175–183

Kosoko O, Sommer A, Auer C 1986 Screening with automated perimetry using a threshold-related three-level algorithm. Ophthalmology 93: 882–886

Krakau C E T, Holmin C 1987 The effect of argon laser trabeculoplasty (ALT) on the visual field decay. In: Kriegelstein G K (ed) Glaucoma update III. Springer-Verlag, Berlin, pp 202–207

Langerhorst C T, Van den Berg T J T P, Greve E L 1989a Fluctuation and general health in automated perimetry in glaucoma. In: Heijl A (ed) Perimetry update 1988/89. Kugler & Ghedini, Amsterdam, pp 159–164

Langerhorst C T, Van den Berg T J T P, Greve E L 1989b Is there general reduction of sensitivity in glaucoma? Int Ophthalmol 13: 31–35

Lewis R A, Johnson C A 1985 Early detection of glaucomatous damage. 1: Psychophysical disturbances. In: Waring G O (ed) Viewpoints. Surv Ophthalmol 30: 111–115

Mikelberg F S, Drance S M 1984 The mode of progression of visual field defects in glaucoma. Am J Ophthalmol 98: 443–445

Mundorf T, Zimmerman T J, Nardin G F et al 1989 Automated perimetry, tonometry, and questionnaire in glaucoma screening. Am J Ophthalmol 108: 505–508

Perimetric Standards and Perimetric Glossary of the International Council of Ophthalmology 1979. Enoch J M (ed). Junk, The Hague

Perkins E S 1973 The Bedford glaucoma survey. 1: Follow-up of borderline cases. Br J Ophthalmol 57: 179–185

Portney G L, Krohn M A 1978 The limitations of kinetic perimetry in early scotoma detection. Ophthalmology 85: 287–293

Quigley H A 1985 Early detection of glaucomatous damage. In: Waring G O (ed) Viewpoints. Surv Ophthalmol 30: 117–128

Quigley H 1989 The optic nerve in glaucoma: lecture presented at the Glaucoma Group Meeting, November 1989, London

Quigley H A, Addicks E M 1982 Quantitative studies of retinal nerve fibre layer defects. Arch Ophthalmol 100: 807–814

Quigley H A, Addicks E M, Green W R 1982 Optic nerve damage in human glaucoma III. Arch Ophthalmol 100: 135–146

Quigley H A, Dunkelberger G R, Green W R 1989 Retinal ganglion cell atrophy correlated with automated perimetry in human eyes with glaucoma. Am J Ophthalmol 107: 453–464

Schmeisser E T, Smith T J 1989 High-frequency flicker visual evoked potential losses in glaucoma. Ophthalmology 620–623

Sommer A, Pollack I, Maumenee E 1979 Optic disc parameters and onset of glaucomatous field loss. Arch Ophthalmol 97: 1444–1448

Traverso C E, Tomey K F, Fatani R 1987 Octopus visual field examination in Saudi Arabia: an assessment of patient performance. In: Greve E L, Heijl A (eds) 7th International visual fields symposium. Doc Ophthalmol Proc Ser. Nijhoff/Junk, Dordrecht 49: 569–575

Tuulonen A, Nagin P, Schwartz B et al 1987 Increase of pallor and fluorescein-filling defects of the optic disc in the follow-up of ocular hypertensives measured by computerized image analysis. Ophthalmology 94: 558–563

Wanger P, Persson H E 1987 Pattern-reversal electroretinograms and high-pass resolution in suspected or early glaucoma. Ophthalmology 94: 1098–1103

Werner E B, Adelson A, Krupin T 1988 Effect of patient experience on the results of automated perimetry in clinically stable glaucoma patients. Ophthalmology 95: 764–767

Wilensky J T, Joondeph B C 1984 Variation in visual field measurements with an automated perimeter. Am J Ophthalmol 97: 328–331

Wilensky J T, Podos S M, Becker B 1974 Prognostic indicators in ocular hypertension. Arch Ophthalmol 91: 200–202

Wu D-C, Schwartz B, Nagin P 1987 Trend analysis of automated visual fields. In: Greve E L, Heijl A (eds) 7th International visual fields symposium. Doc Ophthalmol Proc Ser. Junk, Amsterdam 49: 175–190

7

Uveitis

J. V. Forrester

INTRODUCTION

As time progresses, so our concepts of pathological mechanisms change. For instance, the original categorization of uveitic disease into granulomatous and non-granulomatous forms was valuable in differentiating different clinical types of uveitis as seen by the slit-lamp biomicroscope, and partly assisted in providing an explanation for the presumptive pathology (Woods 1960). Similar distinctions today are described in relation to acute anterior uveitis and its association with allotypes HLA-B27 (Rothova et al 1984) but this does not tell us much more about the pathogenesis of the disease. In contrast, the recent development of experimental models of endogenous uveitis has considerably enhanced our understanding of the clinical disease.

Probably the clearest pathogenetic distinction we can make in uveitis is whether the disease is restricted to the anterior segment or whether it is predominantly a posterior segment disease with variable 'spill-over' into the anterior segment (Forrester 1990). Anterior uveitis is most frequently an acute, recurrent illness involving the iris and ciliary body and may occur as an HLA-B27 positive or a HLA-B27 negative disease (Brewerton et al 1973, Wakefield et al 1984). Chronic forms of anterior uveitis also occur, as with juvenile seronegative arthritis but are much less common.

Posterior uveitis, by contrast, presents with a bewildering variety of clinical syndromes of markedly different severity and visual consequences. Despite this heterogeneity, many forms of this disease are increasingly recognized as representing part of a spectrum of uveoretinal inflammatory disease (Forrester et al 1990).

The cause of most forms of uveitis is unknown despite many associations with connective tissue disease and infectious disease. Viral illness is commonly implicated in anterior uveitis (Byrom et al 1979) and increasingly in certain forms of posterior uveitis such as that associated with cytomegalovirus and herpetic disease (Jabs et al 1989), but for most forms of uveitis no infectious organisms can be identified. Accordingly, a disturbance of immunoregulation (i.e. autoimmunity) has been suggested as the initiator of many types of uveitis. This is particularly so since experimental models of uveoretinitis, which faithfully mimic the various forms of clinical uveoretinitis, can be induced by several different retinal autoantigens, inoculated into experimental animals at sites distant from the eye (Forrester et al 1990).

Autoimmunity and infectious diseases are, however, not mutually exclusive. Current concepts of autoimmune disease include several possible mechanisms whereby invading microorganisms either incorporate themselves into replicating host cells in such a way as to induce an 'altered self' response, or directly initiate an autoimmune response via cross-reacting anti-idiotypic T or B cells which persist long after the inciting microorganism has been eliminated (Vaughan 1989). Since all immune responses, including autoimmune responses, involve presentation of antigen in combination with HLA antigens, it is clear that certain diseases occur more frequently in patients with certain HLA allotypes.

In this chapter, some of the more recent concepts relating to the pathogenesis of anterior and posterior uveitis are considered. In addition, the value of laboratory testing in uveitis is reviewed, and newer approaches to therapy are described.

CLINICAL ENTITIES

Anterior uveitis

Acute anterior uveitis (AAU) occurs with a yearly incidence of 8.2 new cases per 100 000 (Vadot et al 1984) and is the commonest form of uveitis. Approximately half of those cases are HLA-B27 positive and have ankylosing spondylitis or some similar joint disease (Smiley 1974). Initial studies suggested that clinically HLA-B27 positive AAU could be distinguished by the unilaterality and high protein exudation in such patients, while B27 negative AAU patients were more likely to have mutton-fat keratic precipitates (Miettinen & Saari 1977). Recently, Rothova et al (1987) have confirmed these findings in a study of 144 AAU patients in whom 50 clinical variables were analysed using statistical methods. Significantly different findings in HLA-B27 positive patients were: younger age at onset; male predominance; unilaterality with alternating recurrences; plastic and/or fibrinoid aqueous; absence of mutton-fat keratic precipitates; high ocular complication rate and frequent association with spondyloarthropathies. In both groups of patients persistent posterior synechiae occurred (36% and 15% in the B27 positive and negative cases respectively) and it may therefore be difficult to exclude pars planitis from some of these cases. Despite this caveat, it appears from this comprehensive study that HLA-B27 positive AAU is a separate entity from HLA-B27 negative AAU and the former has a worse visual prognosis.

Chronic anterior uveitis is much less frequent than AAU and most commonly occurs in association with juvenile seronegative arthritis (Spalter 1975). Due to the insidious nature of this inflammatory disorder (the 'white eye' uveitis) the visual consequences of this disease can be severe. The inflammation occurs predominantly as a low-grade cellular infiltrate, with marked flare and relative hypotony. Extensive posterior synechiae with cataract formation and secondary cystoid macular oedema account for the visual loss. The aetiology is obscure.

Chronic anterior uveitis can occur secondary to trauma, especially surgical trauma, and frequently reflects a defective blood–aqueous barrier. Although extensive 'flare' in the anterior chamber may not represent continuing inflammatory activity, there is little doubt that persistence of plasma proteins and inflammatory mediators within the anterior chamber will have a deleterious effect on visual function, e.g. by inducing cystoid macular oedema.

Posterior uveitis

Clinical presentation of endogenous posterior uveitis

Endogenous posterior uveitis includes several discrete clinical entities (see Table 7.1), which at first sight might seem to be unrelated. Pars planitis (intermediate uveitis), for instance, involves predominantly the peripheral retina and vitreous base, and characteristically is associated with vitreous inflammatory cell infiltrates (snowballs) and extensive subretinal chorioretinal infiltrates. Careful examination and fluorescein angiography will, however, show that many of these cases also have signs of peripheral retinal vasculitis, while visual loss is most frequently due to macular oedema, itself usually a manifestation of increased leakage from perifoveal capillaries.

Sympathetic ophthalmitis is characterized by the focal chorioretinal nodules or microgranulomata – the Dalen–Fuchs nodules – which typically accumulate as healed scars within the fundus after a short self-limiting period of active inflammation. Similar nodules are observed in sarcoid uveoretinitis (Chan et al 1987), in Vogt–Koyanagi–Harada disease during the phase of resolution (Inomata & Sakamoto 1989), and in the less well-defined disorder of diffuse choroiditis. They are also frequently the cause of exacerbations of vitritis in cases of 'intermediate' uveitis or pars planitis where one or two small, round, white foci in the equatorial or pre-equatorial fundus may be sufficient to cause symptoms of floaters. They often escape detection, however, because they are short-lived and self-limiting, and may disappear

Table 7.1 Endogenous posterior uveitis: clinical syndromes

Intermediate uveitis	Diffuse uveitis
Pars planitis	Panuveitis
Idiopathic retinal vasculitis	Choroiditis:
Sarcoid retinitis/vasculitis	Discrete
Birdshot choroidoretinopathy	Serpiginous
Behçet's disease	
Vogt–Koyanagi–Harada disease	
Some pigment epitheliopathies	
Acute retinal necrosis	

leaving virtually no trace. When they occur in large numbers as in sympathetic ophthalmitis, less so in sarcoidosis, they have a characteristic appearance on fluorescein angiography during the active phase: hypofluorescent choroidal 'spots' in the early sequence with late hyperfluorescence (Sharp et al 1984). Healed, inactive lesions are overlaid by depigmented retinal pigment epithelium and appear as pigment epithelial defects on fluorescein angiography.

Retinal vasculitis involving the posterior pole may present as an 'idiopathic' disorder or as part of a disease entity such as sarcoidosis, Behçet's disease, multiple sclerosis and systemic lupus erythematosus. The vasculitis may affect small or large vessels, and occurs usually as a phlebitis with retinal haemorrhages. Less frequently, an arteritis and phlebitis occur with widespread retinal infiltrates and ischaemia even to the point of retinal necrosis. Retinal vasculitis rarely occurs in isolation. Careful examination will reveal that chorioretinal infiltrates similar to those in sympathetic ophthalmitis are present. In addition, vitreous inflammatory cells are almost a prerequisite for the differentiation of retinal vasculitis from other retinal vascular thrombotic disorders.

Some forms of endogenous posterior uveitis appear to be predominantly choroidal, such as birdshot choroidoretinopathy, in which the hallmark is the widespread distribution of subretinal focal infiltrates and patches of retinal pigment epithelial atrophy. Others appear to be predominantly retinal, such as retinal vasculitis and acute retinal necrosis; while others still produce mainly infiltration of the vitreous with minimal involvement of the ocular coats.

Some disorders appear to have a clear infectious aetiology, such as herpes simplex-induced acute retinal necrosis, cytomegalovirus retinitis and toxoplasmosis retinochoroiditis, although the evidence for the last has become less compelling in the light of recent data showing no clear serological difference between clinically 'toxoplasma' patients and healthy controls (Kijlstra 1990). Most uveitis syndromes, however, are of unknown aetiology and much of the reported histopathology has been concerned with endstage disease (Lightman & Chan 1989). Immunohistopathological studies have shown that T cells, particularly T helper (CD4 +) cells, and monocytes predominate in many lesions such as the Dalen–Fuchs nodule in sarcoidosis and in sympathetic ophthalmitis (Jakobiec et al 1983). Studies of active retinal vasculitis or pars planitis have not been reported in detail but some interesting studies of choroidal changes have been reported in Vogt–Koyanagi–Harada disease (Inomata 1988). In general, however, the available histological data have supported the concept of an immunologically mediated process in most forms of posterior uveitis. In addition, despite the differences in clinical presentation, most forms of posterior uveitis have four cardinal features: (1) vitreous inflammatory cells and exudate (vitreous haze); (2) focal choroidoretinal infiltrates; (3) retinal vasculitis; and (4) macular oedema. In some forms there may be a greater emphasis on one or more of these features such as retinal vasculitis or, in birdshot choroidoretinopathy, focal chorioretinal infiltrates. In other forms, additional features may be present such as retinal necrosis, exudative retinal detachment (in Vogt–Koyanagi–Harada disease), or subretinal and pre-retinal neovascularization. As will be seen from the discussion below, however, these manifestations represent the spectrum of choroidoretinal responses to an inflammatory stimulus and this limited clinical set of responses is essentially the same whether the stimulus is immunological, the result of a chronic infection, or a combination of the two.

PATHOGENESIS OF ANTERIOR UVEITIS

An infectious aetiology for AAU has long been postulated, and has been given greater credence during the last ten years by its link with ankylosing spondylitis and the HLA-B27 antigen. Recent studies have attempted to explain the association between ankylosing spondylitis and certain infectious enterocolitic diseases by suggesting a cross-reaction between certain epitopes (antigenic sites) on the foreign antigen and joint-associated autoantigen which bind specifically to certain HLA-B27 antigens on articular lining cells (de Castro 1989). Protein crystallographic studies have shown that the HLA Class I antigen contains an antigenic peptide-binding region in a cleft between two α-helical regions on the external domains of the α_1- and α_2-chains on its extracytoplasmic surface (Bjorkman et al 1987) (Fig. 7.1). Single amino acid point mutations within the variable region of this binding cleft account for the different allotypes of HLA-B27 (there are seven) and each of these types has variable binding affinity for antigenic peptide and/or the T cell receptor. It has been suggested that the binding cleft of the HLA antigen is normally occupied by (non-immunogenic) autoantigen but, if this site were occupied by cross-reacting or competing foreign peptide, then an immune response might be elicited by presentation of the peptide to the appropriate sensitized cytotoxic lymphocytes which recognize the peptide–MHC antigen complex.

In the case of ankylosing spondylitis, associations have been detected with various infectious diseases, including *Klebsiella* and *Yersinia* enterocolitis and with Reiter's syndrome (Eastmond et al 1980, McGuigan et al 1980, Kuberski et al 1981). Similarly in AAU, association with faecal carriage of *Klebsiella* (White et al 1984) and with recent *Yersinia* infection (Wakefield et al 1990) has been reported, although there is still considerable controversy concerning these results (Kiljstra et al 1986).

There is, however, abundant documented and undocumented clinical evidence for an association of enteric and similar infections with AAU and ankylosing spondylitis. The increasingly convincing laboratory data and the incontrovertible association with HLA-B27 generally support a pathogenetic mechanism in AAU requiring an infectious agent, a genetically susceptible host and autosensitized cross-reactive cytotoxic lymphocytes which target the appropriate peptide–MHC Class I antigen complex on the host cells in both

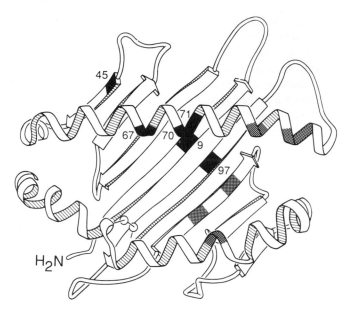

Fig. 7.1 Diagrammatic representation of the MHC Class I antigen, showing the peptide-binding groove between the α_2-chains of the Class I antigen. (With permission, Elsevier publications.)

the eye and the joint, and induce inflammation by damaging these cells. A simpler mechanism for the induction of AAU during infectious states has been proposed which involves release of endotoxin by the invading micro-organisms. This is based on the experimental model of endotoxic uveitis induced in rats by intradermal injections of shigella toxin (Rosenbaum et al 1980). However, this fails to account for the genetic susceptibility of AAU patients and for the delay between development of enteric disease and the later onset of uveitis.

The mechanisms proposed above for HLA-B27 positive AAU do not explain the inflammatory response in the AAU patient who is HLA-B27 negative, or the chronic uveitis in seronegative patients with connective tissue disease. From the clinical presentation it is clear that these patients have a different type of disease, possibly involving different cell types (mutton-fat keratic precipitates (KPs) are more likely to be aggregates of macrophages while fine KPs are probably T lymphocytes) (Rothova et al 1987). In some of these patients, autoimmunity to connective tissue matrix components, such as cartilage and vitreous Type II collagen or proteoglycan, has been proposed. In a model of adjuvant arthritis, in which subcutaneous injections of Freund's complete adjuvant induce a rheumatoid arthritis-like condition (Steffan & Wick 1971) 60% of the animals develop an acute anterior uveitis (Waksman & Bullington 1960). Even in this form of disease, however, infectious agents have been implicated via a molecular mimicry model whereby cross-reaction between a mycobacterial component in the adjuvant and a component in the cartilage proteoglycan has been proposed (Cohen 1988).

The emerging concept, therefore, with regard to AAU is that, while microorganisms, autoimmune or immune-mediated responses, and inflammatory destructive disease are inextricably entwined via processes such as molecular mimicry, the precise mechanisms involved vary significantly between HLA-B27 positive disease and HLA-B27 negative connective-tissue associated disease, and that this distinction probably has important implications with regard to sequelae of the disease (Rothorva et al 1987).

PATHOGENESIS OF POSTERIOR UVEITIS

Despite the marked clinical heterogeneity of posterior uveitis syndromes, information derived from experimental models has greatly assisted us in defining these disorders. Experimental allergic uveoretinitis (EAU) was originally described by Wacker & Lipton (1965) when they used crude extracts of retinal tissue to induce an organ-specific retinal and choroidal inflammation after a single inoculation. Since then, several retinal antigens have been described, including retinal S-antigen, interphotoreceptor retinolbinding protein (IRBP) and even (rhod)opsin itself (Wacker et al 1977, Gery et al 1986, Broeckhuyse et al 1984), each with the ability to induce EAU. Considerable information is now available concerning the amino acid sequence and secondary structure of these proteins (Shinohara et al 1988, Borst et al 1989, Kuhn 1984) and more recently immunodominant epitopes on these antigens have been described at least for retinal S-antigen (Donoso et al 1987) and IRBP (Sanui et al 1989). Despite the lack of sequence homology between these proteins, they all induce a spectrum of EAU severity which can be modified not so much by the nature of the antigen but by the dose of antigen, the species and strain of experimental animal, and the state of immunosuppression of the animal (Forrester et al 1990). Thus low-dose antigen in a low responder rat strain may produce a few focal microgranulomata (similar to Dalen–Fuchs nodules) and minimal evidence of retinal vasculitis (Fig. 7.2), while high-dose antigen will produce extensive destruction of the photoreceptor layer, severe thrombotic retinal vasculitis, exudative retinal detachment and even retinal necrosis (Fig. 7.3) (Forrester et al 1990). Clinically these two extremes might be represented by intermediate uveitis (pars planitis) and acute Vogt–Koyanagi–Harada disease.

The mechanism of the inflammatory response in EAU is currently under intensive investigation. EAU has many similarities with other experimental models of autoimmune disease such as experimental allergic encephalomyelitis (EAE) induced by myelin basic protein and experimental allergic thyroiditis (EAT) induced by thyroglobulin (Alvord et al 1984, Weigle 1980). These diseases, including EAU, are generally induced via activation of CD4 + (T helper) cells and EAU can be transferred by CD4 + cells to naive recipients (Mochizuki et al 1985). In addition, as in human uveitis, there is

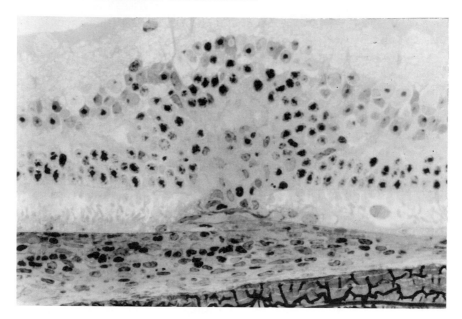

Fig. 7.2   Focal Dalen–Fuchs type nodule in guinea pig EAU.

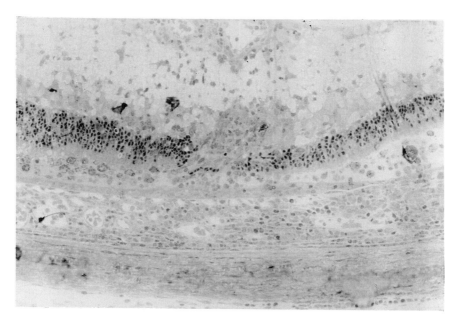

Fig. 7.3   Retinal vasculitis and exudative detached retina in rat EAU.

considerable genetic variability in susceptibility to the disease (Caspi et al 1988), which further emphasizes the importance of the MHC antigen in disease induction.

Generation of an immune response requires processing of antigen (proteolysis) by antigen-presenting cells (APC) and presentation of antigenic fragment(s) (immunogenic peptide) bound to cell surface MHC antigens to the responding T cell. CD4 + (T helper) cells are activated by antigenic peptide bound to MHC Class II molecules on the APC, while CD8 + (T cytotoxic) cells are activated by antigen–MHC Class I complexes (Fig. 7.4). MHC Class II antigens are normally expressed only on 'professional' APC such as macrophages and dendritic cells in lymph node and skin, but tissue cells may be induced to express MHC Class II antigens aberrantly during inflammation (Bottazzo et al 1986). Ocular tissue cells such as retinal pigment epithelial cells, ciliary body epithelial cells, retinal and choroidal vascular endothelial cells (Kusada et al 1989, Fujikawa et al 1987, Liversidge et al 1988) may be induced to express Class II antigens and other 'activation' markers such as the interleukin-2 receptor. Similar findings have been observed in other systems such as the thyroid (Hanafusa et al 1983) and the pancreas (Dean et al 1985) and it has been suggested that aberrant expression of MHC Class II antigen may perpetuate, if not initiate, the autoimmune response (Bottazzo et al 1989). However, this remains a highly controversial area in immunology and, indeed, the opposite mechanism has even been suggested in that expression of Class II antigen, particularly certain forms of DP and DQ antigen in humans, may down-regulate the local immune response (Mitchison 1988).

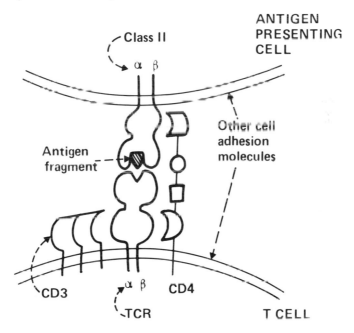

Fig. 7.4   Diagrammatic representation of the molecular interaction between the antigen-presenting cell and the CD4 + (T helper) cell. Accessory molecules include ICAM-1 and LFA-1; CD2 and LFA-3 (see text).

The role of the antigenic peptide in activating the T cell receptor (TcR) has also been extensively studied. Only about 10% of any protein has the capacity to induce an immune response, and identification of immunogenic and uveitogenic sequences on both S antigen and IRBP has been achieved (Donoso et al 1988, 1989). Indeed, dissociation of lymphocyte proliferation sequences and uveitogenic sequences has been observed for S antigen (Gregerson et al 1989, Knospe et al 1988), while specific immunodominant regions of IRBP have been detected (Sanui et al 1989). It is likely, therefore, that the precise way in which the antigen is degraded (processed) by the APC to yield specific fragments will have considerable effect on whether or not an immune response is eventually elicited.

Many questions arise from these studies. For instance, is there a minimal size of peptide required to induce an immune response? Why are some peptides good inducers while others are not? Is the relative affinity of the peptide for the MHC antigen important and is this reflected in genetic susceptibility to disease? Recent studies on peptides from retinal S-antigen have suggested that there is 'core sequence' within the protein which is essential for disease induction and that this sequence has considerable homology for certain sequences from viral and fungal proteins (Singh et al 1990). Indeed, immunization of animals with peptide sequences from baker's yeast has induced an ocular inflammation similar to EAU (Singh et al 1989). If these results are confirmed, they would provide the strongest evidence yet for the molecular mimicry hypothesis involving cross-reactive antigens.

There are many other questions which relate to the pathogenesis of uveitis apart from the activation of sensitized lymphocytes. Two of these concern the mechanism of access of sensitized lymphocytes to the retina, and the role of cytokines in the recruitment of cells to the site of injury and in the process of tissue destruction itself. Homing or accumulation of cells at sites of tissue inflammation has been shown to involve specific cell surface molecules, some of which are important as accessory molecules of adhesion during the interaction between the APC and the T lymphocytes (see Fig. 4.4). Of particular importance are the leucocyte functional antigen LFA-1 and LFA-3 molecules which are distributed on leucocytes and lymphocytes, and the intercellular adhesion molecules, ICAM-1 and ICAM-2, which are also present on circulating lymphocytes but may be expressed on other cell types such as endothelial cells during inflammation (Dustin & Springer 1988, 1989). The ligands for LFA-1 on the endothelium are ICAM-1 and ICAM-2, and for LFA-3 the CD2 molecule on the lymphocyte (Dustin & Springer 1988, 1989, Selvaraj et al 1987). Recruitment of inflammatory cells to sites of retinal injury involves breakdown of the blood–retina barrier at both the vascular endothelium and the retinal pigment epithelium (RPE). Recent studies have shown that in the unstimulated state retinal pigment epithelium cells (RPE) constitutively express ICAM-1 (Fig. 7.5) whereas retinal endothelial cells require trace amounts of interferon-γ to exhibit a high frequency of ICAM-1 antigen (Table 7.2). Neither cell type expressed LFA-1

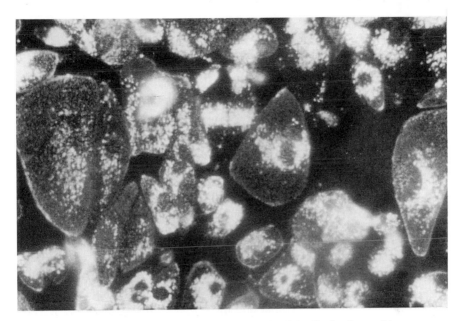

Fig. 7.5 Freshly isolated human retinal pigmented epithelial cells showing positive fluorescence with antibodies to ICAM-1. (Courtesy Dr J. Liversidge.)

antigen or the p150,95 antigen, but a proportion of both RPE cells and endothelial cells expressed the CR3 (Mac-1, CD11b) antigen, a marker for macrophages, suggesting that further complex intercellular interactions with these cells was possible.

In functional terms, expression of these surface molecules on both RPE and endothelial cells was associated with increased adhesion of activated but not resting CD4 + (T helper) cells in vitro (Singh et al 1989, Liversidge et al 1990), and these results suggest that expression of these molecules on cells of the blood–retina barrier may act as the first step in trapping activated T cells at sites of injury. In the presence of specific retinal antigen, local clonal

Table 7.2 Accessory molecule expression by normal and IFN-γ stimulated RPE and EC antigen positive cells (%)

	RPE			EC		
IFN-γ u/ml	0	5 u[a]	500 u[b]	0	5 u[a]	500 u[b]
Monoclonal antibody						
W6/32 (Class 1)	50	100	100	25	100	100
HLA DR	0	0	67	0	0	47
HLA DQ	0	0	46	0	0	51
CD54 (ICAM-1)	81	82	100	18	82	86
CD58 (LFA-3)	0	0	0	100	NT	NT

[a] Cells stimulated with 5 u/ml IFN-γ for 4 hours.
[b] Cells stimulated with 500 u/ml IFN-γ for 4 days.
NT, Not tested.

expansion of the trapped T cells would ensue, with the formation of a small microgranuloma or perivascular infiltrate of cells, as is seen in both EAU and human uveitis. Similar roles for adhesion molecules have been observed in other systems (Dustin & Springer 1988, 1989).

Expression of adhesion molecules and other markers of cell 'activation', such as MHC Class II antigen and the IL-2 receptor, requires local cytokine production at least on endothelial cells. Cytokines such as interferon-γ, tumour necrosis factor and the interleukins (IL-2 to IL-8) have a major role in the initiation and development of the T cell proliferative response (Durum & Mealey 1990). In addition, chemo-attraction of cytotoxic cells such as macrophages, killer cells and cytotoxic T cells, all of which are ultimately the cells which cause tissue damage, is dependent on cytokine production, initially at least by CD4 + cells. Few studies of cytokine production in uveitis have as yet been performed but these factors are undoubtedly produced by T cell lines which induce EAU (Lightman et al 1989) and could offer one avenue of possible therapeutic intervention if their production could be regulated in some way.

Pathogenetic mechanisms in posterior uveitis are therefore highly complex, involving several different cellular and molecular pathways. For each type of posterior uveitis, however, it is likely that the mechanisms are qualitatively similar and that quantitative differences are reflected in the clinical severity and/or pattern of uveitic disease. This offers hope for a logical and uniform approach to immuno-intervention.

LABORATORY TESTING IN UVEITIS

Laboratory testing in uveitis can be considered in four categories: (1) a search for a specific uveitogenic, presumably infectious agent; (2) detection and diagnosis of an underlying systemic disease; (3) determination of genetic susceptibility, e.g. via HLA status; and (4) demonstration of disturbed immunoregulation. While historically there has been enthusiasm for the full 'uveitis screen', in general this has proved unhelpful in the individual case and is not now normally undertaken.

Specific infectious agents

Despite the association between enteric infections, Reiter's arthritis and AAU, faecal and urine cultures are not usually performed in the absence of symptoms of severe prolonged diarrhoeal illness or chronic genitourinary symptoms. Although serological tests have recently shown a strong correlation of AAU with *Yersinia* infection, as yet there is no recommendation that these should be routinely performed since a positive test does not necessarily imply active infections requiring treatment (Wakefield et al 1990). Similarly, viral studies in AAU have shown that a recent infection is not uncommon (Witmer 1972), but such investigations are not of value in the individual case unless there are specific clinical indications (Witmer 1972).

Viral studies in posterior uveitis may be indicated when the clinical appearance of the disease suggests the diagnosis, as in cytomegalovirus retinitis or herpes simplex or herpes zoster-associated acute retinal necrosis. Such cases, however, are relatively uncommon. In addition, serological studies may be relatively uninformative and a definitive diagnosis may require ocular fluid or tissue samples. Analysis of paired serum and aqueous samples for the presence of specific antibodies using commercially available ELISA kits has greatly facilitated diagnosis in these cases, and indicates local intraocular antibody production (Kiljstra 1990).

The most frequently performed test for an infectious agent in posterior uveitis is the toxoplasma serology or dye test. Recent studies, however, have shown that although a negative test is valuable in indicating the absence of previous exposure to the toxoplasma parasite, a positive test does not indicate active disease since a significant proportion of the normal population also have positive tests. Only when a positive serological test is combined with a similarly positive aqueous sample can a definitive diagnosis be made (Kiljstra 1990). The most reliable diagnostic test for toxoplasmosis, therefore, is the fundoscopic appearance. Similar observations apply to tests for presumed ocular histoplasmosis (Schlaegel 1983) and possibly to toxocariasis (Tabbarra 1986).

Detection of underlying connective tissue disease

Many connective tissue diseases have been associated with uveitis. Sarcoidosis can be detected by measuring the serum angiotensin-converting enzyme and serum lysozyme levels (Baarsma et al 1987), and this has a good predictive value. Measurement of autoantibodies to various tissue components such as anti-DNA and anti-smooth muscle are generally unhelpful (Murray 1986), except in cases of juvenile chronic anterior uveitis in which anti-nuclear antibodies may be raised prior to the onset of the joint disease. Patients with symptoms or signs of other systemic disease such as multiple sclerosis, systemic lupus erythematosus or rarer disorders such as Wegener's granulomatosis-like diseases should have appropriate clinical and laboratory tests as indicated. In the last case, testing for anti-neutrophilic cytoplasmic antibody may be valuable (Young et al 1990).

Genetic susceptibility to uveitis

Certain individuals who are particularly susceptible to various forms of uveitis may benefit from HLA phenotyping, particularly if the uveitis occurs in isolation or prior to the onset of systemic signs. For instance, patients with severe, plastic AAU who are found to be HLA-B27 positive will have an increased risk of developing ankylosing spondylitis or Reiter's syndrome (see above). In other cases of uveitis, determination of HLA status may have a diagnostic value, e.g. in cases of suspected birdshot retinochoroidopathy which is linked to the HLA-A29 antigen in over 90% of cases. In most other forms of uveitis, HLA status has little practical value, although it contributes to epidemiological research, for instance, in differentiating racial subtypes of HLA-B5 and B51 positive Behçet's patients.

Immunological tests in uveitis

There have been many studies of various immunological parameters in uveitis. Initial studies of T and B cell subtype populations in AAU and endogenous posterior uveitis suggested that there may be differences between patients and controls (Nussenblatt et al 1980a, Boone et al 1976). However, these have not been confirmed (Froebel et al 1989). In addition, early studies suggesting that there was evidence of specific autoimmunity to retinal antigens (Gregerson et al 1981, Nussenblatt et al 1980b), either by autoantibody testing or in assays of cell-mediated immunity, have also not stood up to further critical analysis (Forrester et al 1989, Doeckes et al 1987, Hirose et al 1988). It is now apparent that most healthy individuals have low levels of antibody to retinal antigens and also have circulating autoreactive T lymphocytes. Indeed, it has been suggested that high levels of anti-retinal antibodies may be protective against the more severe forms of endogenous uveitis (Forrester et al 1989, Dumonde et al 1982), and that in cases of active sympathetic ophthalmitis and Behçet's disease anti-retinal antibodies may be decreased. These results are not unexpected since only a very small proportion of serum immunoglobulins are actually autoreactive, and an even smaller proportion will be specific for retinal antigens. In order to register a significantly positive result, therefore, clonal expansion of specifically sensitized lymphocytes would have to reach extremely high levels.

Recently, markers for 'activated' lymphocytes have become available, including the MHC Class II antigen and the IL-2 receptor. Patients with endogenous uveitis have greater numbers of 'activated' lymphocytes in their circulation than normal individuals (Deschennes et al 1988) and this would coincide with the concept of activated lymphocytes gaining access to ocular tissues by their increased initial adhesiveness to the cells constituting the blood–retinal barrier (see above). Some of these cells are likely to be specific for tissue antigens released during inflammation, and this would stimulate local clonal proliferation at these sites.

Other tests of immune function which have been studied in uveitis include serum immune complexes (Andrews 1979) and complement. In general, testing for immune complexes has not been informative partly because the tests have been applied randomly to many types of uveitis, and partly because of the considerable variability in results for immune complexes. Patients with severe retinal vasculitis have been shown to have reduced levels of immune complexes compared to patients with mild retinal vasculitis (Dumonde et al

1982), but these results have not been confirmed by other laboratories. In addition, there is little pathological or experimental evidence implicating immune complexes in the pathogenesis of retinal vasculitis, which appears to be a T cell-mediated disease.

Detection of low levels of serum complement may suggest immune complex disease due to complement consumption, and occasionally patients with severe retinal vasculitis have been observed with low complement levels (personal observation). However, most cases have normal levels.

In spite of the lack of laboratory evidence supporting an immunological mechanism for the pathogenesis of clinical uveitis, there is little doubt that the disease involves immunological processes in a major if not inciting role. Immunohistologically, ocular tissue from human uveitis cases contains various T cell subsets. In addition, clinical uveoretinitis shows extensive similarity to experimental autoimmune uveoretinitis, induced by recognized autoantigens. Lastly, many forms of endogenous uveitis respond preferentially to immunosuppressants.

CURRENT THERAPEUTIC CONCEPTS

Apart from those rare cases in which a specific aetiological infectious agent has been identified (such as herpetic, cytomegalovirus, *Toxoplasma* or *Toxocara* uveoretinitis), the mainstay of therapy of AAU and endogenous posterior uveitis is immunosuppression. Most cases of AAU will respond adequately to topical steroids (drop, subcutaneous, sub-tenon's or orbital floor), with mydriatics to prevent iris–lens and iris–angle adhesions. Endogenous posterior uveitis also responds well to steroids but usually requires systemic administration to achieve effect.

Steroids, however, and other immunosuppressants such as azathioprine, chlorambucil and cyclophosphamide, are relatively non-specific, and have considerable side effects relating not only to their anti-mitotic effects but to direct toxic effects of the drugs themselves.

The recent introduction of more specific immunosuppressants, such as the CD4+ (T helper) cell inhibitor cyclosporin A (CsA), has added a new dimension to the treatment of steroid-resistant or intolerant cases of sight-threatening uveoretinitis. Experimentally (Nussenblatt et al 1987) and clinically (Nussenblatt et al 1983, Towler et al 1989), CsA is extremely effective in reducing the ocular inflammatory response and in restoring visual function. Initial studies employed CsA at a dose of 10 mg/kg weight and higher, but this was soon found to be nephrotoxic (Palestine et al 1986). CsA-induced renal damage took several forms, including glomerular damage, proximal tubular damage and interstitial fibrosis. In addition, studies of CsA therapy in various forms of transplantation indicated that several other major and minor side-effects were possible (Thiru 1989), although these are much less common in autoimmune disease (von Graffenried et al 1989).

Recent studies of low-dose CsA (Towler et al 1989, 1990) at <5 mg/kg starting dose have shown that the drug is still effective in the treatment of uveitis. Even at this dose, some patients developed renal dysfunction which was, however, partially reversible on reducing the dose further, or stopping the drug altogether. Renal toxicity appeared to be closely linked to the development of hypertension, and this was found to be a useful predictor of the risk of nephrotoxicity (Towler et al 1990). In those patients in whom nephrotoxicity persisted, better control of the inflammatory disease was achieved by combining CsA with low-dose prednisolone and/or azathioprine, while control of the hypertension was best achieved with an angiotensin converting enzyme (ACE) inhibitor. Future developments in this area relate to some of the newer immunosuppressants, such as FK506, an inhibitor of CD4+ cells with an activity similar to CsA but at lower doses. FK506 is effective in inhibiting EAU in various animal models including monkeys (Kawashima et al 1988, Fujimo et al 1990). In liver and renal transplant patients, FK506 has been shown to be remarkably free of nephrotoxicity (Thomson 1990), but studies in autoimmune disease have not yet been initiated. Other macrolide immunosuppressants such as rapamycin may also have potential in the therapy of autoimmune uveitis.

Alternative approaches to immunotherapy relate more closely to the pathogenesis of the disease and the autoantigens which induce them. In experimental allergic encephalomyelitis, a disease similar in pathogenesis to EAU and induced by the central nervous system protein, myelin basic protein (Alvord et al 1984), specially synthesized peptides have been developed which block the binding site for autoantigens on the MHC molecule of the antigen-presenting cell (Urban et al 1989, Wraith et al 1989). Similar approaches could be adopted in EAU but their application to human uveitis is less likely, since the appropriate autoantigen(s) for the human disease have yet to be clearly identified (see above). Indeed, it is highly likely that more than one antigen with more than one immunodominant epitope is implicated in human uveitis. The same reservations, therefore, probably apply to the use of monoclonal antibody therapy in uveitis, although this has been shown to be effective in EAU with antibodies directed against the antigen (Dua et al 1989) or via an anti-idiotypic mechanism (De Kozak et al 1990).

A more direct approach may be to interfere with the function of 'activated' lymphocytes, either by preventing their adhesion to the vascular endothelium as has been shown using antibodies to ICAM-1 (Wegner et al 1990) or by inhibiting the production or function of cytokines released by these activated cells.

We are entering an exciting era in uveitis research both in our understanding of the mechanisms involved in the inflammatory response, in our better recognition of clinical subtypes based on pathogenetic mechanisms and in our approach to therapy. Furthermore, it is likely that the insights gained from this area of research will be applicable generally to the study of autoimmune disease.

REFERENCES

Alvord E C Jr, Keis M W, Suckling A J (eds) 1984 Experimental allergic encephalomyelitis: a useful model for multiple sclerosis. Liss, New York

Andrews G G 1979 Circulating immune complexes in acute uveitis: a possible association with the histocompatability complex locus antigen B27. Int Arch Allergy Appl Immunol 58: 313

Baarsma G S, La Hey E, Glausius E, De Bries J, Kiljstra A 1987 The predictive value of serum angiotensin converting enzyme and lysosyme levels in the diagnosis of ocular sarcoidosis. Am J Ophthalmol 104: 211–217

Bjorkman P J, Sayer M A, Samraoui B, Bennett W S, Strominger J L, Wiley D C 1987 The foreign antigen binding site and T cell recognition regions of class 1 histocompatability antigens. Nature 329: 506–572

Boone W B, Giusta S, Hansen J, Good R A 1976 Lymphocyte subpopulation in patients with sympathetic ophthalmitis and non-granulation uveitis. Invest Ophthal 15: 957–995

Borst D F, Redmond T M, Elser J E et al 1989 Interphotoreceptor retinoid-binding protein. (IRBP): characterisation, protein repeat structures and its evolution. J Biol Chem 264: 1115–1119

Bottazzo G F, Todd I, Mirakian R, Belfiore A, Pujol-Borell R 1986 Organ-specific autoimmunity: a 1986 overview. Immunol Rev 94: 37–169

Bottazzo G F, Bosi E, Bonifacio E, Mirakian R, Todd I, Pujol-Borrell R 1989 Br Med Bull 45: 37–57

Brewerton D A Caffrey M, Michalls A, Walters D, James S C O 1973 Acute anterior uveitis and HLA-27. Lancet ii: 994–996

Broeckhuyse R M, Winkens II J, Kuhlmann E D, van Vugt A H M 1984 Opsin-induced experimental autoimmune retinitis in rats. Curr Eye Res 3: 1405–1412

Byrom M A, Campbell M A, Hobbs J R et al 1979 T and B lymphocytes in patients with acute anterior uveitis and ankylosing spondylitis, and in their household contacts. Lancet ii: 601–603

Caspi R R, Roberge F H, Chan C-C et al 1988 A new model of autoimmune disease. J Immunol 140: 1490–1495

Chan C-C, Metzig R, Palestine A, Kuwabara T, Nussenblatt R B 1987 Immunohistopathology of ocular sarcoidosis. Arch Ophthalmol 105: 1398–1402

Cohen I R 1988 The self, the world and autoimmunity. Sci Am 258: 34–40

Dean B M, Walker R, Bone A J, Baird J D, Cooke A 1985 Prediabetes in the spontaneously diabetic BB/E rat: lymphocyte subpopulations in the pancreatic infiltrate and expression of Class II molecules in endocrine cells. Diabetalalugia 28: 464–466

de Castro J A L 1989 HLA.B27 and HLA-A2 subtypes: structure, evolution and function. Immunol Today 10: 239–246

De Kozak Y, Mirshahi M, Boucheix C, Faure J P, Letts L G, Rothlein R 1990 Prevention of experimental autoimmune uveoretinitis by active immunisation with autoantigen-specific monoclonal antibodies. J Immunol 17: 541–547

Deschennes J, Char D H, Kaliter S 1988 Activated T lymphocytes in uveitis. Br J Ophthalmol 72: 83–87

Donoso L A, Merryman C F, Sery T W et al 1987 S antigen: characterisation of a pathogenic epitope which mediates experimental autoimmune uveitis and pinealitis in Lewis rats. Curr Eye Res 6: 1077–1085

Donoso L A, Yamaki K, Merryman C F, Shinohara T, Yue S, Sery T W 1988 Human S-antigen: characterisation of uveitopathogenic sites. Curr Eye Res 7: 1977–1985

Donoso L A, Merryman C F, Sery T, Sanders R, Vrabec T, Fong S L 1989 Human interstitial retinoid binding protein: a potent uveitopathogenic agent for the induction of experimental autoimmune uveitis. J Immunol 143: 79–83

Doekes G, van der Gaag R, Rothova A et al 1987 Humoral and cellular immune responsiveness to human S antigen in uveitis. Curr Eye Res 6: 909–919

Dua H S, Sewell H F, Forrester J V 1989 The effect of retinal S-antigen specific monoclonal antibody therapy on experimental autoimmune uveoretinitis (EAU) and experimental autoimmune pinealitis (EAP). Clin Exp Immunol 75: 100–105

Dumonde D I, Kasp-Grochowska E, Graham E et al 1982 Anti-retinal autoimmunity and circulating immune complexes in patients with retinal vasculitis. Lancet ii: 787–792

Durum S K, Mealey K 1990 Hilton head revisited: cytokine explosion of the 80s takes shape for the 90s. Immunol Today 11: 103–106

Dustin M L, Springer T A 1988 Lymphocyte function associated antigen-1 (LFA-1) interaction with intercellular adhesion molecule 1 (ICAM-1) is one of at least three mechanisms for lymphocyte adhesion to cultured endothelial cells. J Cell Biol 107: 321–329

Dustin M L, Springer T A 1989 T-cell receptor cross-linking transiently stimulates adhesiveness through LFA-1. Nature 341: 619–624

Eastmond C J, Willshaw H E, Burgess S E P, Shinebaum R, Cooke E M, Wright V 1980 Frequency of faecal *Klebsiella aerogenes* in patients with AS and controls with respect to individual features of the disease. Ann Rheum Dis 39: 118–123

Forrester J V 1990 Endogenous posterior uveitis: a brief review. Br J Ophthalmol 74: 620–623

Forrester J V, Stott D, Hercus K 1989 Naturally occurring antibodies to bovine and human retinal S-antigen: a comparison between uveitis patients and healthy volunteers. Br J Ophthalmol 73: 155–159

Forrester J V, Liversidege J V, Dua H S, Towler H M, McMenamin P G 1990 Comparison of clinical and experimental uveitis. Curr Eye Res 95: 75–84

Froebel K S, Armstrong S S, Urbaniak S J, Forrester J V 1989 An investigation of the general immune status and specific immune responsiveness to retinal S-antigen in patients with chronic posterior uveitis. Eye 3: 263–270

Fujikawa L S, Chan C-C, McAllister C et al 1987 Retinal vascular endothelium expresses fibronectin and Class II histocompatibility complex antigens in experimental autoimmune uveitis. Cell Immunol 106: 139–150

Fujimo Y et al 1990 ARVO abstr. 284–212

Gery I, Mochizuki M, Nussenblatt R 1986 Retinal specific antigens and the immunopathologic process they provoke. Prog Retinal Res 5: 75–109

Gregerson D S, Abrahams I W, Thirkill C E 1981 Serum antibody levels of uveitis patients to bovine retinal antigens. Invest Ophthalmol Vis Sci 21: 669–680

Gregerson D S, Fling S P, Obritsch W F, Merryman C, Donoso L A 1989 Identification of T cell recognition sites in S-antigen: dissociation of proliferative and pathogenic sites. Cell Immunol 123: 427–440

Hanafusa T, Pujol-Borrell R, Chiovato L, Russell R C G, Doniach D, Bottazzo G F 1983 Aberrant expression of HLA-D.R. antigen on thyrocytes in Graves disease: relevance for autoimmunity. Lancet ii: 1111–1114

Hirose S, Tanaka T, Nussenblatt R B et al 1988 Lymphocyte responses to retinal-specific antigens in uveitis patients and healthy subjects. Curr Eye Res 7: 393–403

Inomata H 1988 Necrotic changes of choroidal melanocytes in sympathetic ophthalmia. Arch Ophthalmol 106: 239–242

Inomata H, Sakamoto T 1989 Immunopathological studies of Vogt–Koyanagi–Harada disease with sunset sky fundus. Curr Eye Res 95: 35–40

Jabs D A, Enger C, Bartlett J G 1989 Cytomegalovirus and acquired immunodeficiency syndrome. Arch Ophthalmol 107: 75–80

Jakobiec F, Marboe C, Knowles D et al 1983 Human sympathetic opthalmia. Ophthalmology 90: 76–95

Kawashima H, Fujimo T, Mochizuki M 1988 Effects of a new immuno-suppressive agent, FK 506, on experimental autoimmune uveoretinitis in rats. Invest Ophthalmol Vis Sci 29: 1265–1271

Kiljstra A 1990 Immunological testing in uveitis. Eye (in press)

Kiljstra A, Luyendijk L, van der Gaag R et al 1986 IgG and IgA immune response against *klebsiella* in HLA-B27 associated anterior uveitis. Br J Ophthalmol 70: 85–88

Knospe V, Donoso L A, Banga J P, Yue S, Kasp E, Gregerson D S 1988 Epitope mapping of bovine retinal S-antigen with monoclonal antibodies. Curr Eye Res 7: 1137–1147

Kuberski T T, Morse H G, Ratu R G, Bonnell M D 1981 Increased recovery of *Klebsiella* from the gastrointestinal tract of Reiter's syndrome and ankylosing spondylitis patients. Arthritis Rheum 24 (suppl 1, abstr 123): 78

Kuhn H 1984 Interaction between photoexcited rhodopsin and light-activated enzymes in rods. Prog Retinal Res 3: 123–156

Kusada M, Gaspari A A, Chan C-C, Gery I, Katz S I 1989 Expression of Ia antigen by ocular tissues of mice treated with IFN-gamma. Invest Ophthalmol Vis Sci 30: 764–768

Lightman S, Chan C-C 1989 Immunopathology of ocular inflammatory disorders. In: Lightman S (ed) Immunology of eye diseases. Kluwer, London, pp 87–89

Lightman S, Caspi R, Nussenblatt R 1989 Lymphokine secretion by a CD4 + uveitogenic T-cell line. Invest Ophthalmol Vis Sci 30: 278

Liversidge J, Thomson A W, Sewell H F, Forrester J V 1988 Cyclosporin A, EAU and major histocompatibility Class II antigen expression on cultured retinal pigment epithelial cells. Trans Proc 20: 163–169

Liversidge J, Sewell H F, Forrester J V 1990 Interaction between lymphocytes and cells of the blood–retina barrier: mechanisms of T lymphocyte adhesion to human retinal capillary endothelial cells and retinal pigment epithelial cells in vitro. Immunology 71: 390–396

McGuigan L E, Prendergast J K, Gecgy A F, Edmonds J P, Baskin H V 1980 Significance of non-pathogenic cross-reactive bowel flora in patients with ankylosing spondylitis. Ann Rheum Dis 45: 566–571

Miettinen R, Saari M 1977 Clinical characteristics of familial acute anterior uveitis. Can J Ophthalmol 12: 1–8

Mitchison N A 1988 Suppressor activity as a composite property. Scand J Immunol 28: 271–276

Mochizuki M, Kuwabara T, McAllister C, Nussenblatt R B, Gery I 1985 Adoptive transfer of experimental autoimmune uveoretinitis in rats. Invest Ophthalmol Vis Sci 26: 1–9

Murray P 1986 Serum antoantibodies and uveitis. Br J Ophthalmol 70: 266–268

Nussenblatt R B, Cevario S J, Gery I 1980a Altered suppressor cell activity in uveitis. Lancet ii: 722–723

Nussenblatt R B, Gery I, Ballintine E J, Wacker W B 1980b Cellular immune responsiveness of uveitis patients to retinal S-antigen. Am J Ophthalmol 89: 173–179

Nussenblatt R B, Palestine A G, Chan C-C 1983 Cyclosporin A therapy in the treatment of intraocular inflammatory disease resistant to systemic corticosteroids and cytotoxic agents. Am J Ophthalmol 96: 275–282

Nussenblatt R B, Rodrigues M M, Walker W B et al 1987 Cyclosporin A inhibition of experimental autoimmune uveitis in Lewis rats. J Clin Invest 67: 1228–1231

Palestine A G, Austin H A, Balon J E et al 1986 Renal histopathological alteration in patients treated with cyclosporine for uveitis. N Engl J Med 314: 1293–1298

Rosenbaum J T, McDevitt H O, Guss R B, Egbert P R 1980 Endotoxin-induced uveitis in rats as a model for human disease. Nature 286: 611–613

Rothova A, Kiljstra A, Buitenhuis H J, van der Gaag R, Feltkamp T E W 1984 HLA B27 associated uveitis: a distinct clinical entity? In: Saari K M (ed) Uveitis update. Elsevier, Amsterdam, pp 91–95

Rothova A, van Veenendal W G, Linssen A, Glausius E, Kiljstra A, de Jong P T V M 1987 Clinical features of acute anterior uveitis. Am J Ophthalmol 103: 137–145

Sanui H, Redmond T M, Kotake S et al 1989 Identification of an immunodominant and highly immunopathogenic determinant in the retinal interphotoreceptor retinoid-binding protein (IRPB). J Exp Med 169: 1947–1960

Schlaegel T F 1983 Presumed ocular histoplasmosis. Clin Ophthalmol 4: 1–19

Selvaraj P, Plunkett M L, Dustin M, Sanders M E, Shaw S, Springer T A 1987 The T
    lymphocyte glycoprotein CD2 binds the cell surface ligand LFA-3. Nature 326: 400–402
Sharp D C, Bell R A, Patterson E, Pinkerton R M H 1984 Sympathetic ophthalmia:
    histopathologic and fluorescein angiographic correlation. Arch Ophthalmol 102: 232–235
Shinohara T, Dietschold B, Craft C M et al 1988 Primary and secondary structure of bovine
    retinal S antigen (48K protein). Proc Natl Acad Sci USA 84: 6975–6979
Singh V K, Yamaki K, Donose A, Shinohara T 1989 Molecular mimicry: yeast histone
    H3-induced experimental autoimmune uveitis. J Immunol 142: 1512–1517
Singh V K, Hanspreet K K, Kumihiko Y, Tohru A, Donoso L A, Shinohara T 1990
    Molecular mimicry between a uveitopathogenic site of S-antigen and viral peptides. J
    Immunol 144: 1282–1287
Smiley W K 1974 The eye in juvenile rheumatoid arthritis. Trans Ophthalmol Soc UK 94:
    817–820
Spalter H F 1975 The visual prognosis in juvenile rheumatoid arthritis. Trans Am
    Ophthalmol Soc 73: 544–550
Steffan C, Wick G 1971 Delayed hypersensitivity reaction to collagen in rats with
    adjuvant-induced arthritis. 2. Immunodatsforsh 141: 169–180
Tabbarra K F 1986 Other parasitic infections. In: Tabbarra K F, Hydink R A (eds) Infections
    of the eye. Little, Brown & Co, Boston, pp 679–695
Thiru S 1989 Pathological effect of cyclosporin A in clinical practice. In: Thomson A W (ed)
    Cyclosporin: mode of action and clinical application. Kluwer, Dordrecht, pp 324–364
Thomson A W 1990 FK506 enters the clinic. Immunol Today 11: 35–36
Towler H M, Cliffe A M, Whiting P H, Forrester J V 1989 Low dose cyclosporin A therapy
    in chorionic posterior uveitis. Eye 3: 282–287
Towler H M, Whiting P, Forrester J V 1990 Combination low-dose cyclosporin A and steroid
    therapy in chronic intraocular inflammation. Eye 4: 514–520
Urban J L, Horvath S J, Hood L 1989 Autoimmune T cells: immune recognition of normal
    and variant peptide epitopes and peptide-based therapy. Cell 59: 257–271
Vadot E, Barth E, Billet P 1984 Epidemiology of uveitis: preliminary results of a prospective
    study in savoy. In: Saari K M (ed) Uveitis update. Elsevier, Amsterdam, pp 13–16
Vaughan J H 1989 Infections and autoimmunity. Curr Opinion Immunol 1: 708–717
von Graffenried B, Friend D, Shand H, Schiess W, Timonen P 1989 Cyclosporin A
    (Sandimmun) in autoimmune disorders. In: Thomson A W (ed) Cyclosporin: mode of
    action and clinical application. Kluwer, Dordrecht, pp 213–251
Wacker W B, Lipton M M 1965 Experimental allergic uveitis: homologous retina as
    uveitogenic antigen. Nature 206: 253–258
Wacker W B, Donoso L A, Kalsow C M, Yankeelov D T 1977 Experimental allergic uveitis:
    isolation, characterisation and localisation of a soluble uveitopathogenic antigen from
    bovine retina. J Immunol 119: 1949–1958
Wakefield D, Easter J, Penny R 1984 Clinical features of HLA.B27 anterior uveitis. Aust NZ
    J Ophthalmol 12: 191–196
Wakefield D, Stahlberg T H, Toivanen A, Granfors K, Tennant C 1990 Serologic evidence of
    Yersinia infections in patients with anterior uveitis. Arch Ophthalmol 108: 219–221
Waksman B H, Bullington S J 1960 Studies of arthritis and other lesions induced in rats by
    injection of mycobacterial adjuvant. Arch Ophthalmol 64: 751–761
Wegner C D, Gundel R H, Reilly P, Haynes M 1990 Intercellular adhesion molecule-1
    (ICAM-1) in the pathogenesis of asthma. Science 247: 456–459
Weigle W O 1980 Analysis of autoimmunity through experimental models of thyroiditis and
    allergic encephalomyelitis. Adv Immunol 30: 159–273
White L, McCoy R, Tait B, Ebringer R 1984 A search for Gram negative enteric
    micro-organisms in acute anterior uveitis: association of Klebsiella with recent onset of
    disease, HLA.B27 and B7 CREG. Br J Ophthalmol 68: 750–755
Witmer R 1972 Etiology of uveitis. Ann Ophthalmol 4: 619–628

Woods A C 1960 Modern concepts of the aetiology of uveitis. Am J Ophthalmol 50: 1170–1175

Wraith D C, Similek D E, Mitchell D J, Steinman L, McDevitt H O 1989 Antigen recognition in autoimmune encephalomyelitis and the potential for peptide-mediated immunotherapy. Cell 59: 247–255

Young D W, Dring S, Thompson R A 1990 Anti-neutrophil cytoplasmic antibodies in uveitis. Eye (in press)

8

Cryotherapy of retinopathy of prematurity

A. R. Fielder

INTRODUCTION

The demise of retinopathy of prematurity (ROP) was confidently forecast in the early 1950s and even considered to have already occurred with such definitive statements as 'the flow of blind premature babies ceased like the turning of a tap, and an important cause of blindness was eliminated' (Law 1975). Ophthalmologists are now well aware that unfortunately these hopes proved over-optimistic and blindness induced by ROP is still with us. There have been many references over the past few years to what are now known as the two epidemics of ROP; the first occurring in the 1940s and early 1950s and which was brought to an abrupt end by the discovery that supplemental oxygen was a causative factor. The second epidemic has become apparent over the past decade or so and it is generally attributed to the increased survival of the most immature preterm neonate rather than to new factors (Valentine et al 1989). To support this impression, during the first epidemic the survival of infants of birthweight under 1000 g was about 8% (Silverman 1980). By 1978 this had risen to 48% (Mutch 1986), but has since increased further and is now of the order of 60%. For infants of birthweight under 1500 g survival is about 73% (OPCS 1988).

While improved survival may in part explain the current high incidence of ROP it provides no insight into the basis of the first epidemic. The changing pattern of ROP-related blindness has been carefully documented in a Canadian study undertaken by Gibson et al (1989, 1990). These workers showed that during the 1950s the infants most at risk of blindness from ROP were in the 1000–1500 g birthweight group, but is now mainly confined to those of birthweight 750–999 g, who previously were unlikely to survive. Interesting conclusions can be drawn from this study. First, advances in neonatal management have made an impact on ROP and reduced the risk of blindness for neonates over 1000 g birthweight – important evidence for those who consider ROP an inevitable, and entirely non-preventable consequence of prematurity. Second, although suspected for some time this is documentary evidence of a second epidemic (Gibson et al 1989, 1990, Valentine et al 1989). Third, the first epidemic of ROP, which was largely brought to an end by oxygen restriction, in retrospect could now be called the preventable phase, whereas the second epidemic is currently not preventable. However, in view of the complexities of the management of the extremely immature neonate, preventable and non-preventable ROP may coexist.

The long-term objective is to prevent premature birth, but this not on the immediate horizon. It is important in the meantime to investigate treatment modalities which might lessen or even eliminate the adverse outcome of this still potentially blinding condition.

RETINAL ABLATIVE TREATMENT FOR ROP: THE EARLY PERIOD

By the mid-1960s clinicians realized that ROP was not solely of historical interest. It could not be entirely prevented by either the restriction of oxygen therapy or the ophthalmoscopic monitoring of retinal vessel calibre (Patz 1967, Cantolino et al 1971). Thus in the absence of adequate preventative measures the next logical step was to treat the retinopathy once it had developed. Although primarily concerned with cryotherapy in this chapter, the history of retinal ablative therapy for ROP commenced with photocoagulation, which needs to be considered in this review. Nagata et al in 1967 (Nagata et al 1968) were the first to attempt treatment of severe acute ROP and used xenon arc photocoagulation on one case — 'with dramatic success'. Not surprisingly this prompted a flurry of clinical studies, particularly in Japan using either xenon photocoagulation (e.g. Nagata et al 1968, Oshima et al 1971, Nagata & Tsuruoka 1972, Yamamoto & Tabuchi 1976, Harris & McCormick 1977, Nagata 1977, Koerner 1978), argon laser (Payne & Patz 1972), or cryotherapy (O'Grady et al 1972, Payne & Patz 1972, Yamashita 1972, Sasaki et al 1976, Harris & McCormick 1977, Kingham 1978, Koerner 1978).

Using the criteria of active proliferative disease, progression on follow-up, and significant vitreous haemorrhage, Payne & Patz (1972) treated three eyes with either argon laser or trans-scleral cryotherapy. Provided the ophthalmoscopic view was adequate they considered argon laser the preferred mode, but recommended that until the efficacy of retinal ablative therapy had been established treatment of only one eye per infant was advisable. Yamashita (1972) treated eight cases with cryotherapy and considered this a safe, simple and economic method. Sasaki et al (1976) performed cryotherapy on 16 infants, which they considered was successful in 15 as these eyes only sustained a maximum cicatricial grade 1 or 2. In his introduction to a symposium on ROP in Japan in 1977, Tsukahara pointed out that although photocoagulation and cryotherapy had been performed on many occasions, these methods of treatment should still be considered experimental and long-term verification was required. As most cases of acute ROP undergo spontaneous resolution he recommended future control studies. At that same meeting Uemura (1977) produced on behalf of the Committee for the Study of Retrolental Fibroplasia in Japan guidelines for treatment, recommending photocoagulation for stage 3 acute ROP and active ('rush') circumferential disease. Favourable results following both photocoagulation and cryotherapy were published including the relatively large series of 87 cases by Nagata (1977) and 143 cases by Takagi (1978). Nagata considered that in order to prevent the cicatricial changes of ROP developing, a combination of oxygen curtailment and timely use of retinal photocoagulation was necessary. To achieve this he treated over 21% of infants, and Yamamoto & Tabuchi (1976) 30% of infants of birthweight ≤1500 g. He recognized that this regime inevitably involved the unnecessary treatment of many infants in whom ROP would have undergone spontaneous resolution. Koerner (1978) performed either photocoagulation or cryotherapy on a group of 22 infants. In his opinion, only early and moderate disease was amenable to intervention, and cryotherapy was the preferred mode, although in this study there was no major benefit in the treated compared to the control eye. Keith (1982) performed cryotherapy on nine babies with stage 3 acute ROP which did not appear to influence outcome, whilst Mousel & Hoyt (1980) were cautiously optimistic by stating that treatment may be useful in carefully selected cases. This view was supported by Stark et al (1982), who suggested intervention only for cases where retinal detachment had already occurred. Hindle (1986a, 1986b) treated 30 eyes at either stage 3 or 4 acute ROP. This author applied the cryoprobe to the ridge–extraretinal fibrovascular proliferative complex, and reported that in order to minimize adverse consequences treatment must be undertaken before severe stage 3 is established. It is pertinent to note that all reports quoted so far applied treatment to the vascularized ridge and in some cases this also extended posteriorly (Stark et al 1982), anteriorly and posteriorly (Mousel & Hoyt 1980), or anteriorly onto the avascular peripheral retina (Nagata 1977). Harris & McCormick (1977) attempted to evaluate four treatment methods: photocoagulation (1) to the retina posterior to the ridge, (2) to the ridge itself; and cryotherapy (3) to the ridge or (4) to the ridge and anterior avascular retina. Not surprisingly on a group of only 12 infants it was not possible to differentiate the effects of these treatment types. Nagata (1977) considered coagulation of the ridge to be most effective but postulated that treatment to the avascular retina might also be appropriate by decreasing mesenchymal complexes and their contribution to the subsequent proliferative response. He later modified this view, recommending treatment to the avascular zone alone, and that cryotherapy directly applied to the newly formed vessels or the retina posterior to the ridge is contraindicated (quoted by Ben-Sira & Nissenkorn 1986).

Ben-Sira & Nissenkorn (1980) were the first to confine treatment consistently to the avascular retinal zone, deliberately avoiding the neovascular ridge. They treated 18 eyes which had progressed beyond stage 2 acute ROP with subsequent 'good' vision in 15 of these eyes. These data were updated in 1986 (Ben-Sira & Nissenkorn) to 39 cases. None progressed beyond stage 2 cicatricial disease and in their opinion cryotherapy removed the danger of complete blindness. At between five and eight years post-treatment, visual function was good, with only a few anatomical abnormalities (Nissenkorn et al 1983). Compared to ex-preterms who had no, or mild (stage 2) ROP, the treatment group had more myopia and astigmatism, although in this study the effects of prematurity, ROP and cryotherapy could not be completely differentiated. Tasman (1985) also treated the avascular retina in 17 eyes. Although 71% of treated compared to 41% of untreated eyes improved, numbers were too small to reach significance. However, a continuation of this study (Tasman et al 1986) permitted the inclusion of a further 11 eyes ($n = 28$), by which time it was demonstrated that cryotherapy was significantly preferable to no treatment ($p < 0.001$). Topilow & Ackerman (1989) treated the avascular region of 50 eyes of 25 infants, and while in all the neovascularization regressed, 11 eyes went on to retinal detachment. Bert et al (1981) combined cryotherapy with scleral buckling. However, this procedure was only performed at an advanced stage when retinal detachment had already developed. Retinal reattachment was achieved in all seven treated eyes.

Although the treatment for severe ROP started using photocoagulation, this was superseded by cryotherapy, this mode being more effective and easier to deliver to the infant eye. Perhaps more important than the mode are three other aspects: the site, extent and timing of treatment. Most early studies applied treatment directly to the ridge, although in some this also extended posteriorly, anteriorly (Harris & McCormick 1977), or on both sides (Tamai 1986); indeed some authors recommended applying treatment to the avascular zone, particularly if wide (Uemura 1977, Nagata & Tsuruoka 1972). Nagata (1977) and later Ben–Sira & Nissenkorn (1986) showed that treating the avascular area alone was effective and less likely to cause complications, such as haemorrhage. The early retinal ablative literature contains little precise information on the extent of treatment, although Yamashita (1972), Sasaki et al (1976) and Tamai (1986) all considered that it was only necessary to apply treatment to a few discontinuous areas such as a maximum of four spots per retinal quadrant. Others including Sasaki (1976) and Hindle (1986a, 1986b) confined treatment to the area of fibrovascular proliferation. Ben-Sira et al (1980) and Tasman (1985) treated the full circumference of the avascular area, the latter author taking care to avoid freezing the area of fibrovascular proliferation itself. Yamamoto & Tabuchi (1976) appreciated the dilemma, stating that treatment should be neither too early nor too late, yet acknowledging that the decision to intervene is difficult in a rapidly progressive condition. As mentioned, due to the absence of an agreed classification before 1984, critical analysis of those studies undertaken before that time and direct comparison with current practice is not possible. For this reason many clinical details have been largely ignored. Nevertheless it is apparent that in many of the early studies the timing of treatment was undertaken when the acute process was over, the process of contraction of the fibrovascular elements had already commenced, and further contraction was inevitable; i.e. treatment was at best likely to be ineffective but more likely to be harmful (Ben-Sira &

Nissenkorn 1986). In contrast, a few workers treated eyes at an earlier stage than would now be considered necessary (Nagata 1977, Ben-Sira et al 1980).

The absence of an internationally agreed classification for ROP prevented the comparison of findings between centres and was recognized as a major hindrance to progress in clinical ROP research and hence the management of this condition. It was the driving force which led to the formation of the Committee for the Classification of Retinopathy of Prematurity and the publication of the International Classification of acute ROP in 1984 (Table 8.1) and the late stages in 1987. This proved to be highly significant in the history of the study and management of this condition and scientifically important, for it recognized the importance of both location of the retinal lesion by retinal zone (centred on the optic disc), and its extent of involvement in each zone by clock hour (Table 8.1). Of great practical importance for clinicians was its ease of use and the simplicity of recording findings. For the first time in the history of ROP, direct comparison between centres became possible and heralded an appropriate time to reconsider the role of

Table 8.1   International classification of retinopathy of prematurity

Stage	
1	*Demarcation line*: thin line, within the plane of the retina separating avascular from vascular retinal regions
2	*Ridge*: the line of stage 1 has increased in volume and extends out of the plane of the retina. Isolated vascular tufts may be seen posterior to the ridge, but are not stage 3
3	*Ridge with extraretinal fibrovascular proliferation*, which may be: (i) Continuous with the posterior ridge edge (ii) Posterior, but disconnected, from the ridge (iii) Into the vitreous
4	*Retinal detachment — subtotal* A Extrafoveal B Retinal detachment involving the fovea

5	*Retinal detachment — total*
	Funnel: *Anterior* *Posterior*
	          open open
	          narrow narrow
	          open narrow
	          narrow open

'Plus' disease: iris vascular engorgement and rigidity, dilatation, tortuosity and engorgement of retinal vessels, vitreous haze. These are in addition to the signs above: signs of activity

Location of ROP
Zones — centred on optic disc:
Zone 1   From disc to twice macular disc distance — 30°
Zone 2   To ora serrata nasally, extends in a circle around the anatomical equator. Temporally not simple to identify precisely
Zone 3   Anterior to zone 2, is present temporally, inferiorly and superiorly, but not nasally

Extent of ROP: recorded as clock hours in each eye
Regressed ROP: primarily concerned with the management of stage 3, and the later phases will not be considered here

cryotherapy for severe disease. Only three of the aforementioned studies (Hindle 1986a, 1986b, Tasman et al 1986, Topilow & Ackerman 1989, 1990) postdate this event, therefore direct comparison between current practice and many of the earlier studies is not appropriate, and for this reason precise clinical details have not been presented.

The importance of this pioneering clinical work must not be underestimated, and to be entirely dismissive would be to ignore an inevitable preliminary process which enabled subsequent progress in the management of severe ROP. Taking an overall view of these studies it is apparent that treatment by either photocoagulation or cryotherapy did sometimes halt the progress of severe ROP and hasten its resolution but they were inconclusive, due to problems of classification, a paucity of data and insufficient patient numbers. They did, however, provide the stimulus for further investigation. By the 1980s the second epidemic was well under way and it became imperative to determine whether retinal ablative therapy was effective for acute ROP. With an internationally acceptable classification the time was now appropriate for a multicentre trial of cryotherapy for ROP.

THE MULTICENTRE TRIAL OF CRYOTHERAPY FOR RETINOPATHY OF PREMATURITY

To attempt to overcome the problems outlined above, Drs Flynn and Palmer in the USA developed the idea of a multicentre trial for cryotherapy (Spencer 1990). Due to its impact on current practice, it will be considered here in detail.

The primary aim of this randomized study was to determine prospectively whether cryotherapy is efficacious in the treatment of severe acute ROP. The secondary aim was to study the natural history of this condition. Because of the possible harm of cryotherapy, only one eye of each infant was treated.

Study design and patient groups (CRPCG 1988)

The study design has been discussed in detail by Palmer et al (1985) and Spencer (1990). In brief, infants of birthweight ≤1250 g who were without a major congenital anomaly were potentially eligible for inclusion in the study. Twenty-three centres participated with enrolment of infants, commencing January 1986. After the initial ophthalmic examination undertaken between 28 and 42 days after birth, conditional upon gaining parental consent, the infant was enrolled into the natural history group of the cryotherapy study. Those with either no, or mild ROP (less than pre-threshold), were examined on a fortnightly basis until retinal vascularization was complete.

The natural history group

As described, the entire cohort of neonates was included in the natural history group, of which a subgroup became eligible for entry into the randomized study group. This cohort was examined on a fortnightly basis until retinal vascularization was complete, and then reviewed at 3, 12 and 24 months, corrected ages. This group contained those without, and those with, the milder stages of ROP, but who did not reach the pre-threshold stage. Infants who developed pre-threshold disease were examined at weekly intervals until the process had regressed to below the pre-threshold, or threshold ROP occurred (see Table 8.2 and Fig. 8.1 for details of pre-threshold and threshold). The results of the natural history group have yet to be published.

The randomized study group

At threshold ROP in one or both eyes, the infant was entered, again dependent upon parental consent, into the randomized study group (late enrolment was also possible at this stage for babies from non-participating centres suspected of having threshold disease). Infants with both eyes reaching threshold ROP simultaneously (symmetrical) were randomly assigned for one eye to receive cryotherapy, with the other eye acting as control. For those with only one eye at threshold (asymmetrical), treatment was randomly assigned for that eye. If this resulted in no treatment being given, in the event of the second eye later progressing to threshold, this eye was treated. The final data analysis did not include the second eye of asymmetrical cases.

Upon randomization, cryotherapy was undertaken within 72 hours, unless in the interim the eye had progressed to stage 4, in which case the eye was excluded. Transscleral cryotherapy, in contiguous but not overlapping applications, was performed to the entire circumference of the avascular retina extending from the ora serrata to the anterior edge of the fibrovascular ridge. Full procedural details will be discussed later.

Preliminary results (CRPCG 1988)

Between 1st January 1986 and 31st October 1987, 9356 neonates of birthweight ≤1250 g had been identified in the 23 centres. For a number of reasons this number was reduced to 3862 by 28 days after birth.

Outcome at three months was judged on anatomical criteria alone, by two methods: stereo photographs of the posterior pole (not including the retinal periphery) and clinical examination. Unfavourable outcome was classified as:

Table 8.2

Pre-threshold ROP
Zone 1   Any stage
Zone 2   Stage 2 with 'plus' disease
        Stage 3   ″   ″   ″

Threshold ROP
5 contiguous or 8 cumulative clock hours stage 3
— in zone 1 or 2, with 'plus' disease

Right   Left

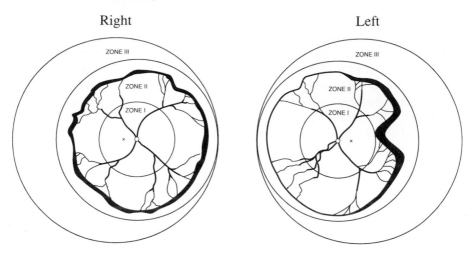

Fig. 8.1   Right eye: zone 2 ROP stage 3 extending to involve about 11 clock hours; left eye: zone 2 ROP stage 3 involving 4 clock hours.

retinal fold across the macula, retinal detachment involving the posterior pole, or total retrolental mass.

This preliminary report presented the results of 172 of the 291 randomized eyes which had completed three months follow-up. The mean birhweight (Bwt) and gestational age (GA) of the randomized group was 800 g and 26.3 weeks, respectively. In 82% the disease was symmetrical between the eyes. The average age at intervention was 11.4 weeks after birth. Photographic assessment revealed unfavourable outcome in 43% of untreated and 21.8% of treated eyes, a reduction of the unfavourable outcome of 49.3% ($p < 0.00001$). Clinical evaluation gave similar results. For untreated eyes asymmetrical disease had a better outcome than symmetrical (unfavourable in 5.3% versus 24.1%, respectively). Thus for those untreated eyes there was an unfavourable outcome in 45.6% with symmetrical, and in 15.4% with asymmetrical disease.

As the risk of unfavourable outcome in severe stage 3 acute ROP was so significantly reduced by cryotherapy (almost 50%), the trial was terminated early, and further randomization ceased. This action was taken due to the committee's concern for the welfare of those neonates at risk, but not falling within the study who might not receive the benefit of treatment.

In conclusion, the authors recommended cryotherapy for at least one eye of threshold symmetrical ROP, while for the fellow eye the clinician's own judgment should be used as to whether this eye should also receive treatment.

Three-month outcome (CRPCG 1990a)

Between 1st January 1986 and 30th November 1987, 9751 neonates were identified, of whom 291 (including 73 late entries) were entered into the randomized study. The mean Bwt and GA of this cohort was 800 g and 26.3

weeks, respectively. By three months corrected age, photographs were available on 260 infants. The unfavourable outcome was reduced by 39.5% ($p < 0.0001$), with the greatest reduction occurring in symmetrical disease (40.6%), and zone 2 (46.3%), compared to zone 1 disease (17.3%). Of those eyes which received cryotherapy, 31% deteriorated to an unfavourable outcome. Ophthalmoscopic and photographic findings concurred.

Thus the findings of the preliminary report on the benefit of cryotherapy were confirmed. In addition, clinical findings also reported benefits of cryotherapy for the whole eye, such as a reduced propensity to develop glaucoma. Despite the poor prognosis of zone 1 disease even after treatment (unfavourable outcome in 94% without, and 78% following treatment), intervention still conferred a degree of benefit and the authors recommended that cryotherapy be considered for both eyes in this group. This article concluded by stating the need for screening programmes in neonatal units.

One-year outcome: structure and function (CRPCG 1990b)

This cohort reviewed at one year corrected age remained unchanged from that at three months. In addition to the photographic and ophthalmoscopic anatomical evaluations undertaken at previous stages of this study, for the first time visual function was quantified using a clinical adaptation of the preferential looking technique: the acuity card procedure. Acuity cards use gratings and will often be referred to as grating acuities.

Of the 291 randomized infants 246 were available at one year. Outcome based on assessment of retinal photographs showed a reduction in unfavourable outcome of 45.8%, compared to the control group, confirmed clinically. Grating acuities were significantly better in the treated compared to the untreated eyes (35.0% versus 56.3%), with 60.0% of the former falling within the normal range, in contrast to only 41.0% of the latter. These results do, however, emphasize the seriousness of ROP, as 50.6% of the controls and 31.9% of the treated eyes fell into the blind or low-vision category.

Thus at one year corrected age the beneficial effect of cryotherapy on severe acute ROP remains and is significant for each birthweight group and also according to the clock hour extent of involvement. The reduction in other ocular abnormalities in the treated compared to the untreated, noted at three months, was also confirmed. Between three and 12 months, ten infants changed favourable/unfavourable status, equal numbers moving in each direction.

The advisability of treating both eyes in zone 1 disease was again stated, but for zone 2 disease has not been established. This dilemma was addressed by Phelps & Phelps (1989), who recommended treating only one eye in moderately severe ROP, but two eyes in cases whose severity rises well above threshold. That the reduction in unfavourable outcome was maintained at one year indicates that the benefits of cryotherapy are likely to be long term.

Thus, 21 years, and many inconclusive studies after Nagata et al (1968) first treated ROP with xenon arc photocoagulation, retinal ablative therapy has been found to have a significant beneficial effect on the retina, the eye as a whole, and most important on visual function. Already the results of this study have had considerable impact on ROP management across the world. The remainder of this chapter will consider the management of severe ROP in the light of this important study.

SEVERE ROP: MANAGEMENT OF THE INFANT AT RISK

At present ROP is not entirely preventable and, as mentioned previously, serious disease can still develop despite meticulous neonatal care. The role of the ophthalmologist has always been less than satisfactory in the past as he or she could neither prevent nor treat this condition. But, with the results from the Multicenter Trial of Cryotherapy this situation has changed. Now for the first time the ophthalmologist can significantly reduce the unfavourable outcome in severe disease. Furthermore, the medicolegal responsibility, which to date has rested predominantly with causation, may well in the future involve ophthalmic management.

Screening for severe ROP

As the infant at risk of developing severe ROP must first be identified, the topic of screening needs to be raised before discussing the technicalities of cryotherapy. The primary purpose of screening is to identify pre-threshold ROP which may progress to threshold disease and require cryotherapy (see review by Urrea & Rosenbaum 1989). The results from the Multicenter Trial have shown that there is only a narrow time window during which treatment can be successfully applied, which in retrospect was not appreciated in many early studies as intervention had often been either too early or too late. Clearly therefore an understanding of the natural history of ROP is a necessary prerequisite to the identification of ROP at an appropriate time to permit intervention.

That the incidence and severity of acute ROP rises with increasing immaturity is well known, and its incidence in infants of birthweight under 1000 g is between 60% and 88% (Keith & Kitchen 1984, Reisner et al 1985, Schaffer et al 1985, Flynn et al 1987, Ng et al 1988). All stage 1 and stage 2 ROP will undergo spontaneous and clinically complete resolution. Certain other aspects of its natural history, such as its age at onset, rate of progression and retinal location, are less well known but are important clinical aids to screening and will now be considered.

Time of onset and progression

ROP cannot develop after completion of retinal vascularisation, just after term. But events before this time are quite intriguing for, while ROP is a condition of the developing retinal vessels, the most immature, often very poorly neonate, does not develop retinopathy until a later postnatal age than his or her less premature counterpart (Fielder et al 1986). Corrected for the degree of prematurity, ROP develops over a relatively narrow postmenstrual age range (surprisingly, the terms for corrected age – postmenstrual, PMA, and postconceptual, PCA – are used synonymously!) and in a recent study 86% ROP developed between 32.5 and 38.5 weeks PMA (Fielder et al 1986). Thus the age at which retinopathy develops (but not its occurrence or severity) is controlled predominantly by the stage of development rather than neonatal events. Once present, its subsequent progression also appears to be predetermined, as shown in Figure 8.2 (Fielder et al 1991). Practically, this is useful information (and theoretically fascinating), for ophthalmic examinations can be planned according to PMA/PCA rather than postnatal age. Furthermore factors such as oxygen treatment or incubation need not influence the timing of examination, although of course the fitness of the baby to undergo this assessment must be taken into account. ROP is rare before 31 weeks PMA; thus a normal examination very early has no screening value,

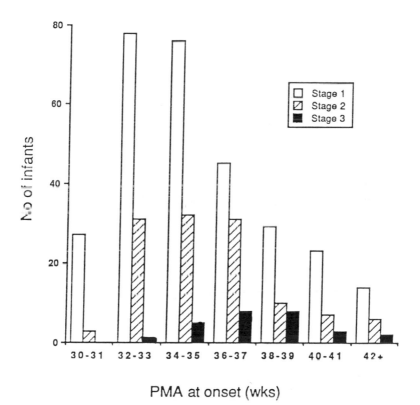

PMA at onset (wks)

Fig. 8.2 Postmenstrual age at onset of ROP and its progression in 572 infants to birthweight ≤1700 g. Note no ROP was observed before the 30th week despite over 200 infants born before this time. For examination protocol see Ng et al (1988).

and a first examination after discharge from hospital may well be too late. Most stage 3 develops between about 34 and 42 weeks PMA, and ROP commencing after 36 weeks is most unlikely to progress further to stage 3.

ROP location

In the first epidemic, ROP was observed to commence in the temporal retina — not surprising as this is the last retinal region to vascularize. But those were relatively more mature than the neonates currently surviving and it has recently been shown that in the most immature neonates ROP commences, preferentially in the nasal retina (Fielder et al 1987, 1988b, 1991). The more posterior the location of ROP, by zone, the greater its propensity to progress to stage 3. This information is of practical value. ROP confined to zone 3 rarely if ever progresses to stage 3, the caveat to this statement being that the examiner must be confident of his or her ability to locate precisely the retinal findings by zone. It is the opinion of this writer (but by implication, not all agree) that an eyelid speculum and scleral indentor are important examination aids, for they permit the rapid and accurate evaluation of peripheral nasal retinal vascularisation, i.e. whether in zone 2 or 3.

These few comments on the natural history of ROP simplify routine screening, and have influenced the drawing up of guidelines recently issued jointly by the College of Ophthalmologists and the British Association for Perinatal Medicine (1990). They recommended the screening of all neonates under 1500 g Bwt and under 32 weeks GA. Examinations for all should commence at 7 weeks postnatal age. For those under 26 weeks GA, examinations should be continued fortnightly until 36 weeks PMA. For those 26–31 weeks GA, after the examination at 7 weeks there should be a final examination at around 36 weeks PMA (the aim being to complete screening before discharge from hospital). Obviously from these guidelines 7 postnatal weeks and 36 weeks PMA for the larger baby may be very close, and one examination will often suffice. Clinical judgment must be used, and the examination protocol should be modified by any ROP that develops.

The cryotherapy procedure

The neonate at risk of developing, or the one who already has, severe ROP, is immature, fragile and frequently very poorly. Without underestimating the importance of the ophthalmic disorder, clearly the general welfare of the infant must be placed foremost and any procedure must be undertaken in collaboration with the neonatologist. Finally, consider the parents who, with their baby, have just passed or are still passing through a highly traumatic period. By the time ROP reaches threshold stage (around 11 weeks after birth; CRPCG 1988, 1990a), hopefully parents are beginning to relax, and are just daring to make firm plans for their baby's future. It does not require much imagination to appreciate the devastating effect the ophthalmologist can have on presenting them with the news, possibly not even suspected, that their infant having survived the traumas of the neonatal period is now at risk of becoming blind.

Timing of cryotherapy

Although, as mentioned, the general status of the infant must be taken into account, the time window for cryotherapy is short, and once threshold ROP has been diagnosed there should be as little delay as possible before proceeding. In the Multicenter Trial of Cryotherapy (CRPCG 1988, 1990a) this was set at a maximum of 72 hours to minimize the risk of further progression, and was performed on average at 11.3 weeks after birth (range 6.6–23.9 weeks), i.e. a mean of 37.7 weeks PMA CRPCG 1990a.

Anaesthesia

Either general or local anaesthesia can be used (Fig. 8.3), and there are no strong factors indicating a preference for one over the other. More important, neonatal medical staff need to be in attendance and involved in the procedure. Facilities for resuscitation must be immediately at hand. For these reasons most procedures are undertaken on neonatal units, and the infant remains an in-patient for at least 24 hours.

If local anaesthesia is used, this can be topical alone, with subconjunctival infiltration, and with or without sedation/analgesia. The procedure is painful

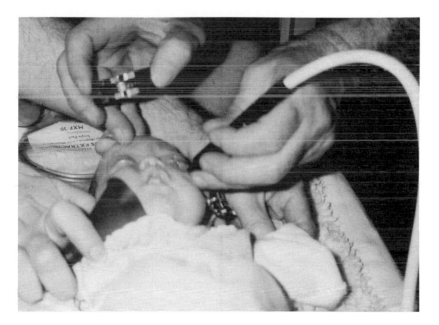

Fig. 8.3 Cryotherapy being performed in a sedated infant.

and this writer utilizes topical anaesthesia with sedation/analgesia. Brown et al (1990) reported respiratory and cardiorespiratory arrest in a few infants who received subconjunctival infiltration of local anaesthesia. While they were unable categorically to identify the cause of this serious complication they recommended: the avoidance of excessive subconjunctival anaesthetic (use appropriate dose for body weight); the use of preoperative administration of systemic atropine to minimize the oculocardiac reflex; analgesia; and the availability of adequate monitoring facilities. Retrobulbar anaesthesia is not recommended as the orbital bones are very thin. A satisfactory approach is to use a combination of topical and systemic anaesthesia/sedation, the latter being administered through an intravenous line, which is kept in place at least during the procedure. Details of the systemic agents have been deliberately omitted as these are for the neonatologist in attendance to prescribe.

Systemic complications encountered during cryotherapy include bradycardia, cyanosis, hypoxaemia and respiratory depression (Brown et al 1990, CRPCG 1990a), but no deaths have been reported.

Cryoapplication

The pupils can be dilated by a variety of topical agents, usually a combination which includes phenylephrine 2.5% (*not* the more concentrated preparation). The procedure is done under direct visualization, using indirect ophthalmoscopy.

A variety of cryotherapy probes have been used: retinal, paediatric or cataract. While narrow-shafted probes facilitate access, the size of the lesion is inevitably smaller and more applications are required. An eyelid speculum is used to gain access to the globe. It is rarely necessary to open the conjunctiva.

The aim of treatment is to produce cryotherapy lesions, which are contiguous but not overlapping, to the avascular retina, i.e. from the ora serrata to the anterior edge of the neovascular ridge, but taking care to avoid the ridge itself. The end point is just at the appearance of a white lesion. Proceeding to further whitening is not necessary and may predispose to haemorrhage. The cryoprobe is applied first to the ora serrata and the entire circumference at this level is treated, followed by the more posterior applications. This sequence softens the globe and facilitates access to its posterior aspects. Usually about 50 applications are necessary (CRPCG 1988).

Postoperative management

Instillation of a mydriatic is recommended for a few days, but unless the conjunctiva has been opened no other topical medication is required. Within 24–72 hours vessel engorgement should begin to subside. The indication for retreatment (not strictly correct, as it is the untreated skip areas which are treated) is the persistence of plus disease 3–17 days after cryotherapy, in the presence of skip areas. Retreatment, which should be undertaken within two to three weeks, is required in about 5% of cases.

Complications

Lacerations and haemorrhage of the conjunctiva can occur (5.3% and 11.7%, respectively; CRPCG 1990a). Retinal, preretinal and vitreous haemorrhage have also been reported (together 22.3%, CRPCG 1990a). Retinal tear has been noted, as has transient occlusion of the central retinal artery (CRPCG 1990a). Greven & Tasman (1989) reported the development of retinal detachment in three eyes more than a year after cryotherapy. Optic atrophy is infrequently noted (Hindle 1986b, CRPCG 1990a), but is probably not a complication of cryotherapy per se, but of neurological damage.

THE CONSEQUENCES OF CRYOTHERAPY

So far, although the major results of cryotherapy have been presented, certain other topics have received little or no attention.

Ocular growth and refractive development

The last few weeks of gestation are particularly active for ocular growth (review, Fielder 1988a) and this process can be retarded by severe ROP (Kelly & Fielder 1987). It is of interest that most of this growth is in the anterior part of the globe and retina: the region over which cryotherapy is applied. Whilst these are early days for evaluating the effects of cryotherapy on the eye, it is gratifying that no reports of inhibition of ocular growth have yet been reported. As an example, this author followed an infant who received cryotherapy to one eye: the corneal diameter of the untreated eye lagged behind the fellow eye, and while the degree of microcornea diminished over a two-year period it was not eliminated.

The association of myopia with cicatricial ROP is well known, and its magnitude is positively correlated with severity (Nissenkorn et al 1983). Eyes which have been subjected to cryotherapy appear to be more myopic than untreated eyes (Ben-Sira & Nissenkorn 1986, CRPCG 1990a), but this finding, or more correctly this deduction, may be in part spurious as the fellow eye may have media opacities, retinal detachment, etc.

Development of visual functions

The difficulty of correlating ophthalmic findings with function is well known, but has recently been restated in the context of the Multicenter Trial of Cryotherapy by Spencer (1990): 'No one disputes that the adverse outcome criteria produce a poor visual result. What is less certain is the effect on vision' and of other less serious consequences.

Grating acuity development has been reported as being normal in the first two years of life in regressed stage 3 ROP (Luna et al 1990), except for those who had neurological abnormalities. Birch & Spencer (1991), however, found that even in infants with regressed ROP and normal posterior poles there was a slight but significant acuity deficit (0.28 octave) compared to normals. These authors also found a strong correlation between anatomical category and visual function. The beneficial effect of cryotherapy on acuity has already been mentioned, with 41.1% untreated, but 60.0% treated eyes falling within the normal range (CRPCG 1990b). Compare these with a group of infants, also from this trial (Quinn et al 1990), who developed retinal detachment and were managed either conservatively (71 eyes) or underwent vitrectomy (58 eyes). Despite anatomical alignment in 28% only two eyes had any measurable pattern vision, and that at the lowest spatial frequency available for testing. These results show that preferential looking-based techniques are now making significant inroads into clinical practice and providing information which hitherto was simply not available. Dobson et al (1990) were able to obtain data from 95% of 1-year-olds with high inter-observer reliability. Peripheral visual field dysfunction, either by delayed development or constriction, has been reported in stage 3 ROP not submitted to cryotherapy, without cicatricial sequelae (Luna et al 1989). There is no information on the influence of cryotherapy on visual field development.

This leads to the final part of this chapter. What should the clinician say to the parents of the patient? A recent leader in the *Lancet* on ROP (Editorial 1991) ended with: 'there is a tendency to neglect the long-term consequences of ROP for affected individuals and their families'. Referring to the first epidemic: 'Most of the parents harboured bitterness towards their doctor, not for failure to anticipate the disastrous effects of oxygen therapy, but for their apparent indifference to their plight. This is an appalling indictment of medical behaviour that the profession cannot ignore.' While cryotherapy has significantly reduced the unfavourable outcome for severe ROP, it is no panacea. These comments forcefully make the point that the ophthalmologists' role extends far beyond the management of the retinal condition, into spheres in which we have little expertise. This cannot be considered further, other than to avoid a defensive approach and for free communication with parents and those involved in the care of the visually impaired child.

But hopefully, the infant with severe ROP who has just received cryotherapy will not be visually impaired. Parents still need to be informed as soon as possible, be it favourable or not. The acuity card procedure permits vision to be measured at frequent intervals from very early infancy (see above). Although there are certain concerns about its comparability with results obtained by a Snellen recognition test, particularly in amblyopia, in the context of the infant who may be visually impaired it is invaluable. It is important that whatever test is used its limitations at that time are appreciated, and inappropriate predictions are not made for the future. For instance acuities obtained at say three, six and nine months of age provide information pertinent for those times *only*. Thus from serial normal acuities the parents can be told that vision lies within normal limits, but one cannot predict that acuity will, or will not, continue to mature at a normal rate. Within these limitations, parents can be kept informed of visual development, be it normal or abnormal, and if the latter given some knowledge of its magnitude early on. While this will not alter management at a retinal level, it does permit the clinician to gain insight into the kinetics of visual recovery, the effectiveness of treatment, and the early organization of support if the child proves to be visually impaired.

To summarize, retinal ablative treatment for ROP commenced in 1967, but it was not until publication of the preliminary results of the first Multicenter Trial of Cryotherapy for Retinopathy of Prematurity in 1988 that the beneficial effects of this treatment mode on severe acute ROP were confirmed. With the increased survival of the very immature neonate the implications of these findings for future ophthalmic practice are considerable.

REFERENCES

Anon 1990 College news: ROP screening duty. Q Bull Coll Ophthalmol (Autumn): 6
Ben-Sira I, Nissenkorn I 1986 Treatment of acute retinopathy of prematurity with cryotherapy: the Beilinson experience. In: McPherson A R, Hittner H M, Kretzer F L (eds) Retinopathy of prematurity. BC Decker, Toronto, pp 129–141
Ben-Sira I, Nissenkorn I, Grunwald E, Yassur Y 1980 Treatment of acute retinopathy of prematurity. Br J Ophthalmol 64: 758–762
Ben-Sira I, Nissenkorn I, Weinberger D et al 1986 Long-term results of cryotherapy for active stages of retinopathy of prematurity. Ophthalmology 93: 1423–1428
Bert M D, Friedman M W, Ballard R 1981 Combined cryosurgery and scleral buckling in acute proliferative retrolental fibroplasia. J Pediatr Ophthalmol Strabismus 18: 9–12
Birch E E, Spencer R 1991 Visual outcome in infants with cicatricial retinopathy of prematurity. Invest Ophthalmol Vis Sci 32: 410–415
Brown G C, Tasman W S, Naidoff M, Schaffer D B, Quinn G, Bhutani V K 1990 Systemic complications associated with retinal cryoablation for retinopathy of prematurity Ophthalmology 97: 855–858
Cantolino S J, O'Grady G E, Herrera J A, Israel C, Justice J, Flynn J T 1971 Ophthalmoscopic monitoring of oxygen therapy in premature infants: fluorescein angiography in acute retrolental fibroplasia. Arch Ophthalmol 72: 322–331
Committee for the Classification of Retinopathy of Prematurity 1984 An international classification of retinopathy of prematurity. Arch Ophthalmol 102: 1130–1134
Committee for the Classification of Retinopathy of Prematurity 1987 An international classification of retinopathy of prematurity. II The classification of retinal detachment. Arch Ophthalmol 105: 906–912
CRPCG (Cryotherapy for Retinopathy of Prematurity Cooperative Group) 1988 Multicenter trial of cryotherapy for retinopathy of prematurity: preliminary results. Arch Ophthalmol 106: 471–479
CRPCG (Cryotherapy for Retinopathy of Prematurity Cooperative Group) 1990a Multicenter trial of cryotherapy for retinopathy of prematurity: three-month outcome. Arch Ophthalmol 108: 195–204
CRPCG (Cryotherapy for Retinopathy of Prematurity Cooperative Group) 1990b Multicenter trial of cryotherapy for retinopathy of prematurity: one year outcome. Arch Ophthalmol 108: 1408–1416

Dobson V, Quinn G E, Biglan A W, Tung B, Flynn J T, Palmer A E 1990 Acuity card assessment of visual function in the cryotherapy for retinopathy of prematurity trial. Invest Ophthalmol Vis Sci 31: 1702–1708

Editorial 1991 Retinopathy of prematurity. Lancet 337: 83–84

Fielder A R, Ng Y K, Levene M I 1986 Retinopathy of prematurity: age at onset. Arch Dis Child 61: 774–778

Fielder A R, Ng Y K, Levene M I, Shaw D E 1987 Retinopathy of prematurity: age at onset and the initial site of involvement: a preliminary report. In: BenEzra D, Ryan S J, Glaser B M, Murphy R P (eds) Ocular circulation and neovascularisation. Martinus Nijhoff/Dr W Junk, Dordrecht pp 147–154

Fielder A R, Moseley M J, Ng Y K 1988a The immature visual system and premature birth. In: Whitelaw A, Cooke R W I (eds) The very immature infant. Br Med Bull 44: 1093–1118

Fielder A R, Ng Y K, Shaw D E, Levene M I 1988b Retinopathy of prematurity: natural history. Invest Ophthalmol Vis Sci 29 (suppl): 121

Fielder A R, Shaw D E, Robinson J, Ng Y K 1991 Retinopathy of prematurity: natural history (submitted)

Flynn J T, Bancalari E, Bachynski B N et al 1987 Retinopathy of prematurity: diagnosis, severity and natural history. Ophthalmology 94: 620–629

Gibson D L, Sheps S B, Schechter M T, Wiggins S, McCormick A Q 1989 Retinopathy of prematurity: a new epidemic? Pediatrics 83: 486–492

Gibson D L, Sheps S B, Uh S H, Schechter M T, McCormick A Q 1990 Retinopathy of prematurity-induced blindness: birth weight-specific survival and the new epidemic. Pediatrics 86: 405–412

Greven C M, Tasman W 1989 Rhegmatogenous retinal detachment following cryotherapy in retinopathy of prematurity. Arch Ophthalmol 107: 1017–1018

Harris G S, McCormick A Q 1977 The prophylactic treatment of retrolental fibroplasia. Mod Probl Ophthalmol 18: 364–367

Hindle N W 1986a Cryotherapy for retinopathy of prematurity: timing of intervention. Br J Ophthalmol 70: 269–276

Hindle N W 1986b Location and timing of intervention with cryotherapy. In: McPherson A R, Hittner H M, Kretzer F L (eds) Retinopathy of prematurity. BC Decker, Toronto, pp 143–149

Keith C G 1982 Visual outcome and effect of treatment in stage III developing retrolental fibroplasia. Br J Ophthalmol 66: 446–449

Keith C G, Kitchen W H 1984 Retinopathy of prematurity in extremely low birthweight infants. Med J Aust 141: 225–227

Kelly S P, Fielder A R 1987 Microcornea associated with retinopathy of prematurity. Br J Ophthalmol 71: 201–203

Kingham J D 1978 Acute retrolental fibroplasia. II. Treatment by cryosurgery. Arch Ophthalmol 96: 2049–2053

Koerner F H 1978 Retinopathy of prematurity: natural course and management. Metab Ophthalmol 2: 325–329

Law F W 1975 The history and traditions of the Moorfields Eye Hospital, Vol II. HK Lewis, London, p 203

Luna B, Dobson V, Carpenter N A, Biglan A W 1989 Visual field development in infants with stage 3 retinopathy of prematurity. Invest Ophthalmol Vis Sci 30: 580–582

Luna B, Dobson V, Biglan A W 1990 Development of grating acuity in infants with regressed stage 3 retinopathy of prematurity. Invest Ophthalmol Vis Sci 31: 2082–2087

Mousel D K, Hoyt C S 1980 Cryotherapy for retinopathy of prematurity. Ophthalmology 87: 1121–1127

Mutch L M M 1986 Epidemiology, perinatal mortality and morbidity. In: Roberton N R C (ed) Textbook of paediatrics. Churchill Livingstone, Edinburgh, pp 3–19

Nagata M 1977 Treatment of acute proliferative retrolental fibroplasia with xenon-arc photocoagulation. Jpn J Ophthalmol 21: 436-459

Nagata M, Tsuruoka Y 1972 Treatment of acute retrolental fibroplasia with xenon arc photocoagulation. Jpn J Ophthalmol 16: 131-143

Nagata M, Kobayashi Y, Fukuda H, Suekane K 1968 Photocoagulation for the treatment of the retinopathy of prematurity. Jpn J Ophthalmol 22: 419-427

Ng Y K, Fielder A R, Shaw D E, Levene M I 1988 Epidemiology of retinopathy of prematurity. Lancet ii 1235-1238

Nissenkorn I, Yassur Y, Mashkowski Y, Sherf I, Ben-Sira I 1983 Myopia in premature babies with and without retinopathy of prematurity. Br J Ophthalmol 67: 170-173

Office of Population Census and Surveys 1988 OPCS monitor

O'Grady G E, Flynn J T, Herrera J A 1972 The clinical course of retrolental fibroplasia in premature infants. South Med J 65: 655-658

Oshima K, Ikui H, Kano M, Nakama T, Kumano S, Hiyoshi Y 1971 Clinical study and photocoagulation of retinopathy of prematurity. Folia Ophthalmol Jpn 22: 700-707

Palmer E A, Biglan A W, Hardy R J 1985 Retinal ablative therapy for active retinopathy of prematurity: history, current status and prospects. In: Silverman W A, Flynn J T (eds) Contemporary issues in fetal medicine and neurology 2. Retinopathy of prematurity. Blackwell, Boston, pp 207-228

Patz A 1967 New role for the ophthalmologist in prevention of retrolental fibroplasia. Arch Ophthalmol 78: 565-568

Payne J W, Patz A 1972 Treatment of acute proliferative retrolental fibroplasia. Trans Am Acad Ophthalmol Otolaryngol 76: 1234-1241

Phelps D L, Phelps C E 1989 Cryotherapy in infants with retinopathy of prematurity: a decision model for treating one or both eyes. JAMA 261: 1751-1756

Quinn G E, Dobson V, Barr C C et al 1990 Visual acuity in infants after vitrectomy for severe retinopathy of prematurity. Ophthalmology 98: 5-13

Reisner S H, Amir J, Shohat M, Krikler R, Nissenkorn I, Ben-Sira I 1985 Retinopathy of prematurity: incidence and treatment. Arch Dis Child 60: 698-701

Sasaki K, Yamashita Y, Maekawa T, Adachi T 1976 Treatment of retinopathy of prematurity in active stage by cryocautery. Jpn J Ophthalmol 20: 384-395

Schaffer D B, Johnson L, Quinn G E, Weston M, Bowen F W 1985 Vitamin E and retinopathy of prematurity. Ophthalmology 92: 1005-1011

Silverman W A 1980 Retrolental fibroplasia: a modern parable. Grune & Stratton, New York

Spencer R 1990 The CRYO ROP study: a national cooperative study of retinopathy of prematurity. In: Eichhenbaum J W, Mamelok A E, Mittl R N, Orellana J (eds) Treatment of retinopathy of prematurity. Year Book Publishers, Chicago, pp 143 168

Stark D J, Manning L M, Lenton L 1982 The incidence and the results of active treatment of acute retrolental fibroplasia. Aust J Ophthalmol 10: 135-140

Takagi I 1978 Treatment of acute retrolental fibroplasia. Ophthalmol Jap 82: 323-330

Tamai M 1986 Treatment of acute retinopathy of prematurity by cryotherapy and photocoagulation. In: McPherson A R, Hittner H M, Kretzer F L (eds) Retinopathy of prematurity. B C Decker, Toronto, pp 151-159

Tasman W 1985 Management of retinopathy of prematurity. Ophthalmology 92: 995-999

Tasman W, Brown G C, Schaffer D B et al 1986 Cryotherapy for active retinopathy of prematurity. Ophthalmology 93: 580-583

Topilow H W, Ackerman A L 1989 Cryotherapy for advanced stage 3 + retinopathy of prematurity: visual and anatomical results. Ophthalmol Surg 20: 864-871

Topilow H W, Ackerman A L 1990 Cryotherapy for advanced stage 3 + retinopathy of prematurity. In: Eichhenbaum J W, Mamelok A E, Mittl R N, Orellana J (eds) Treatment of retinopathy of prematurity. Year Book Publishers, Chicago, pp 125-142

Tsukahara I 1977 Introduction to the symposium: retinopathy of prematurity. Jpn J Ophthalmol 21: 401-403

Uemura Y 1977 Current status of retrolental fibroplasia: report of the joint committee for the study of retrolental fibroplasia in Japan. Jpn J Ophthalmol 21: 366-378

Urrea P T, Rosenbaum A L 1989 Retinopathy of prematurity: an ophthalmologist's perspective. In: Isenberg S J (ed) The eye in infancy. Year Book Publishers, Chicago, pp 428–456

Valentine P H, Jackson J C, Kalina R E, Woodrum D E 1989 Increased survival of low birth weight infants: impact on the incidence of retinopathy of prematurity. Pediatrics 84: 442–445

Yamamoto M, Tabuchi A 1976 Management of the retinopathy of prematurity. Jpn J Ophthalmol 20: 372–383

Yamashita Y 1972 Studies on retinopathy of prematurity III. Cryocautery for retinopathy of prematurity. Jpn J Clin Ophthalmol 26: 385–393

9

Pneumatic retinopexy

D. A. Brinton   G. F. Hilton

INTRODUCTION

Intravitreal gas was first used in 1911 (Ohm 1911). Over the last two decades, its use was developed in conjunction with scleral buckling, drainage of subretinal fluid, and/or vitrectomy (Norton 1973, Escoffery et al 1985).

Hilton & Grizzard (1986) introduced the term 'pneumatic retinopexy' and described the technique of gas injection plus cryopexy or laser for repairing retinal detachment. Since that report, over 100 studies have been published on pneumatic retinopexy including a multicentre randomized controlled clinical trial (Tornambe et al 1989) and statistical reports on 1274 cases. The single-operation success rate in these 1274 eyes is 80%, and 98% were reattached with reoperations, which compares favourably with scleral buckling (Hilton 1990), but the visual results are significantly better with pneumatic retinopexy than with scleral buckling (Tornambe et al 1989).

Pneumatic retinopexy is an alternative to scleral buckling for the surgical repair of selected retinal detachments. A gas bubble is injected into the vitreous cavity, and the patient is positioned so that the bubble closes the retinal break(s), allowing resorption of the subretinal fluid. Laser photocoagulation or cryotherapy is applied around the retinal break(s) to form a permanent seal. The procedure can be done in an outpatient setting, and no cutting of the eye is required.

INTRAOCULAR GASES

Choice of gases

Sulphur hexafluoride (SF_6) is the gas most frequently used with pneumatic retinopexy, followed by perfluoropropane (C_3F_8). Other perfluorocarbon gases are in current use, and success has also been reported with sterile room air.

In selecting a gas, it is important to understand the longevity and expansion characteristics of the gases. SF_6 doubles in volume within the eye, reaching its maximum size at about 36 hours. It will generally disappear within about 10–12 days, depending on the amount injected. Perfluoropropane quadruples in volume, reaching maximum size in about three days. The bubble will last

30–45 days in the eye. Room air does not expand but immediately starts to resorb. The air bubble will be gone within just a few days (Table 9.1).

The choice of type and amount of gas depends on the following considerations.

What size gas bubble is needed?

One must usually plan for a gas bubble large enough to cover all open breaks simultaneously and keep them covered for three to five days, with some extra as a margin of error.

Hilton & Grizzard (1986) did computerized tomographic studies on eyes with intravitreal gas bubbles. These results differed substantially from those obtained by Parver & Lincoff (1977) in model eyes. In the human, a 0.3 ml gas bubble covers about 60° of arc of the retina, but it takes approximately a 1.2 ml bubble to cover 80–90°.

Usually, 0.3–0.6 ml of gas are injected into the eye. If it is desired to inject more than 0.6 ml into the eye, multiple injections should be planned, allowing return of intraocular pressure towards normal between injections.

How long do you want the bubble to stay in the eye?

We feel that it is optimal for the gas bubble to cover the break(s) for five days and then disappear as soon as possible. A lingering gas bubble may induce tears, since movement of the head causes forcible movements of the vitreous when a gas bubble is in the eye.

In most cases, the prolonged longevity of a perfluoropropane bubble is a disadvantage, to be balanced against the advantage of injecting a smaller amount of gas initially.

The longevity of air is probably sufficient for most cases, but sometimes the chorioretinal adhesion may not be sufficiently mature when the air has resorbed. Air also forfeits the advantage of post-injection expansion within the eye. Therefore, air has not generally been our gas of choice.

Because reasonable differences of opinion exist regarding the relative merits of the various gases, a new multicentre randomized controlled clinical trial is addressing the issue of choice of gas. Sulphur hexafluoride is being compared with perfluoropropane. Until these results dictate otherwise, our gas of choice in most cases is SF_6. We use C_3F_8 for the occasional case which

Table 9.1 Intravitreal gas duration and expansion

Gas	Average duration	Largest size by	Average expansion
Air	3 days	Immediate	No expansion
SF6	10 days	36 hours	Doubles
C3F8	35 days	3 days	Quadruples

requires an exceptionally large and long-acting gas bubble to tamponade large or widespread breaks. Most of the time we inject 0.4–0.5 ml of 100% SF_6.

Characteristics of gases

The following characteristics of gases account for their efficacy in reattaching the retina:

1. *Surface tension* allows the gas bubble to occlude a retinal break instead of passing into the subretinal space. The surface tension of any gas is much higher than that of other substances in the eye. Once the break is occluded, the retinal pigment epithelial pump can reabsorb the subretinal fluid.

2. *Buoyancy* provides the force which pushes the uppermost retina back against the wall of the eye. Apposition of the retina against the choroid is necessary in order that chorioretinal adhesion can occur, just as two surfaces to which glue have been applied must be clamped together while the glue dries.

The initial expansion of SF_6 and C_3F_8 is due to the law of partial pressures and the solubility coefficients of the gases involved. A 100% SF_6 bubble injected into the eye contains no nitrogen, oxygen, etc., but these gases are dissolved in the fluid around the bubble. Due to the law of partial pressures, nitrogen and oxygen will diffuse into the gas bubble. SF_6 also starts to diffuse out of the gas bubble into the surrounding fluid which contains no SF_6. However, nitrogen and oxygen diffuse across the gas–fluid interface much more quickly than SF_6 because of the relative insolubility of SF_6. The net result is an initial influx of gas molecules into the bubble, expanding its size until partial pressures equilibrate to the point where net influx equals net egress, and maximum expansion is reached. Then the bubble gradually resorbs as the SF_6 is slowly dissolved in the surrounding fluid. The diameter of the bubble shrinks at an approximately constant rate until the gas is gone. C_3F_8 expands more and reabsorbs more slowly because it is even less soluble than SF_6.

PREOPERATIVE EVALUATION

Good preoperative evaluation is vital to the success of pneumatic retinopexy. Pneumatic retinopexy is not a good procedure for surgeons lacking in excellent retinal examination skills, for two reasons:

1. Scleral buckling with encirclement may achieve retinal reattachment even if a retinal break is missed (Griffith et al 1976). It can be a very 'forgiving' procedure in this sense. With pneumatic retinopexy, it seems that any missed retinal break can open into a detachment. The presence of a gas bubble within the vitreous cavity causes shifting of the subretinal fluid or vitreous which can open previously attached breaks.

2. When scleral buckling is done, the surgeon gets a second look in the operating room with the patient sedated, with full control of the globe, and with open conjunctiva for deep scleral depression. With pneumatic retinopexy, this is not available.

In addition to a thorough examination of the retina, the preoperative evaluation for possible pneumatic retinopexy should include assessment of the following:

1. Is the patient mentally capable of following positioning directions?
2. Is the patient physically capable of maintaining positioning as needed, especially with regard to neck and back problems?
3. Will it be feasible from the standpoint of the patient's home situation for the patient to maintain the appropriate position postoperatively?
4. Will he be able to return to the surgeon's office for frequent follow-up as required?
5. Does the patient have plans to travel in the near future, especially by air, which might pose a hazard with an intraocular gas bubble?
6. Does the patient have evidence of severe glaucoma?
7. Has the patient had recent surgery on this eye which would require care to avoid causing dehiscence of the healing incision?
8. Does the presence of a filtering bleb or a corneal transplant require special handling?
9. Would the induction of increased myopia that generally occurs following an encircling buckle be an advantage or disadvantage given the patient's refractive status?
10. Does the patient's general health contraindicate the use of general anaesthesia for scleral buckling?

Because postoperative patient cooperation is essential, the nature of the procedure and what will be expected of him should be discussed thoroughly with the patient before surgery.

OPERATIVE TECHNIQUE

The technique detailed here is essentially the same as that originally described by Hilton & Grizzard (1986), with a few modifications. The operation is usually done in an outpatient department or in the surgeon's office.

Anaesthesia

Retrobulbar anaesthesia is usually used for pneumatic retinopexy. An injection into the anterior muscle cone will usually produce anaesthesia without akinesia initially. This has the advantage of allowing the patient to position his eye to cooperate with cryopexy. After the retrobulbar anaesthetic is given, cryopexy is administered promptly before the eye becomes akinetic.

Topical anaesthesia, with subconjunctival injection as needed, can be used with some patients, but it does not block the pain and the vagal response which can occur with very high ocular pressure. Rarely, general anaesthesia is indicated because the patient is very apprehensive.

Cryo versus laser

Pneumatic retinopexy is generally done in one session with cryopexy applied to the retinal breaks prior to gas injection. An alternative technique involves a two-part procedure, utilizing laser instead of cryo. The first part of the procedure consists of injection of a gas bubble into the vitreous cavity. The patient maintains appropriate head positioning at home with follow-up in the surgeon's office. Once the break is reattached, laser treatment is applied.

The photocoagulation is greatly facilitated by use of an indirect ophthalmoscopic laser, which makes it easy to position the patient's head to move the gas bubble away from the break(s) (Friberg & Eller 1988). Treatment can also be applied with a slit-lamp laser delivery system by tilting the patient's head as needed.

Alternatively, one can treat the breaks through the gas bubble if the bubble is moderately large. When treating through gas, one must be careful not to overtreat. Gas has an insulating effect, conducting heat away from the laser spot at a slower rate than liquid vitreous, which may result in excessive thermal burns with retinal necrosis and hole formation. Avoid treating close to the edge of the bubble where total internal reflectivity might conceivably result in reflections onto the macula.

Laser treatment can even be applied if the retina is not yet entirely attached. By treating with laser through the gas bubble, the detached tear can be temporarily held in apposition to the wall of the eye while laser is applied.

There is some evidence to suggest that cryopexy is associated with a higher incidence of proliferative vitreoretinopathy and other complications (Campochiaro et al 1985). In addition, the chorioretinal adhesion with laser may be quicker and firmer than that with cryo (Friberg 1989). On the other hand, the one-part procedure with cryo is usually more convenient, and the breaks may be easier to find and treat when they are open. Another multicentre randomized pneumatic retinopexy trial is currently under way, in part to determine whether cryo or laser is the preferable technique.

Certain circumstances might indicate use of laser instead of cryo. If a tear appears to be under considerable vitreous traction, laser might be preferred. If multiple and/or large breaks are present, the risks of extensive cryopexy might warrant the use of laser instead.

Preparing the eye

Following the anaesthetic and cryopexy, the next step is to massage the eye to reduce intraocular volume, making room for the gas bubble. Retropulsion of the eye into the orbit dehydrates the orbital fat but is less effective at reducing the intraocular volume. Instead, a scleral depressor is placed against the temporal equator and the eye is pressed firmly against the bony nasal orbital wall. Firm pressure is applied for 45 seconds, then relaxed for 15 seconds to allow perfusion of the retinal vasculature. This cycle is repeated until the intraocular pressure is less than 5 mmHg. This manoeuvre causes egress of fluid from the eye, but also stretches the scleral fibres, allowing more ample intraocular volume (Schaffer 1985). Examination and cryopexy with firm scleral depression will have started this process, but usually additional massage is needed. Preoperative medication for reducing the intraocular pressure can be used but saves little massaging time, so we have dropped it from the protocol.

A sterile lid speculum is utilized. Undiluted Betadine solution is instilled directly onto the cornea and conjunctiva. After 3 minutes the injection site is dried with a sterile cotton tipped applicator and the eye is ready for injection of gas.

Be certain to use Betadine solution rather than other preparations of Betadine which may contain alcohol or detergent. Preoperative topical antibiotics add nothing to the sterility of a careful sterile preparation. Meticulous sterility is mandatory. No cases of endophthalmitis have been reported following pneumatic retinopexy when Betadine solution was used as described above.

Preparing the gas

A pressure-reducing system is attached to the gas cylinder to allow drawing the gas from a low-pressure system. High pressure can blow out the millipore filter and render it useless in sterilizing the gas (Packo 1989). A condom catheter can be attached to the cylinder, or a step-down valve system can be used. Alternatively, the gas may be transferred to a large syringe and then a small volume is easily transferred to a 3-ml syringe.

The selected gas is drawn through a millipore filter into a 3-ml syringe in sterile fashion. The tube connecting the gas cylinder with the syringe, including the filter, is flushed through with gas to ensure no dilution with room air. Draw a few millilitres of gas into the syringe, discard, and fill the syringe again. A disposable 30-gauge $\frac{1}{2}$-inch (12-mm) needle is then placed tightly on the syringe and excess gas is expelled, to leave the exact amount intended for injection. The gas should not be stored in the syringe for more than a few minutes prior to injection because room air will infiltrate the syringe and dilute the gas sample (Humayun et al 1989).

Injecting the gas

An injection site is selected 3–4 mm posterior to the limbus. Select a site away from large open retinal breaks, highly detached retina, or detached pars plana epithelium. The head of the supine patient is turned to one side to make the injection site uppermost. The needle is then passed into the eye perpendicular to the sclera (Fig. 9.1). Push the needle 6–8 mm into the eye to ensure that the tip is well into the vitreous, directing the tip away from areas of highly bullous detachment. Then withdraw until 3 mm of the needle remains in the eye. This will ensure that the tip remains in the vitreous but is shallow enough to prevent multiple small bubbles ('fish eggs').

A caliper can be used to ensure that the needle is withdrawn to the proper point. Not all $\frac{1}{2}$-inch needles are exactly $\frac{1}{2}$ inch, so measure your needle carefully.

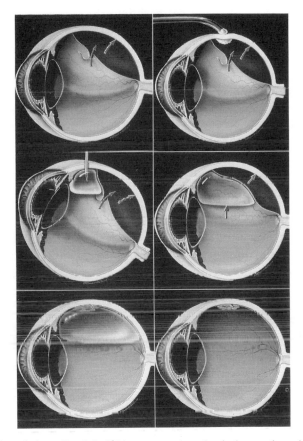

Fig. 9.1 Basic technique. Top left: fluid can enter the subretinal space through the open break (lower arrow) faster than the retinal pigment epithelial pump can resorb it into the choroid (upper arrow). Top right: the area of the retinal break is treated with multiple contiguous applications of transconjunctival cryotherapy. Alternatively, laser treatment is applied later when the retina is reattached. Middle left: with the pars plana injection site uppermost, the gas bubble is injected into the vitreous with a 30-gauge needle. Unless the breaks are small, injection is made away from the area of the breaks. Middle right: the head is positioned so that the intravitreal gas bubble closes the retinal break. If the macula is still attached but threatened, the 'steamroller' manoeuvre is used. Bottom left: with the break closed by the gas bubble, the retina is usually reattached by the first postoperative day. Bottom right: the gas bubble resorbs spontaneously. Reproduced with permission from J. B. Lippincott Company, Journal of Ophthalmology.

We do not recommend trying to visualize the needle tip with an indirect ophthalmoscope. The manoeuvring required to do so may cause the needle tip to damage intraocular structures, and we doubt that the appropriate depth can be more accurately gauged than by external measurement.

With the needle in the correct position, the entire volume of gas is injected briskly. This facilitates formation of a single bubble at the needle tip. The injecton should not be so brisk as to force bubbles of gas deep into the vitreous before their buoyancy can make them rise. Inject smoothly and quickly but not with excessive force. Hold the plunger down until the needle is withdrawn to prevent escape of gas back into the syringe.

We recommend that the patient's head be rotated 90° to the opposite side before withdrawing the needle. This allows the bubble to float away from the injection site and prevents gas from escaping through the needle tract. This manoeuvre should be rehearsed with the patient prior to inserting the needle to ensure smooth coordination. With only 3 mm of the needle in the eye, this manoeuvre has not caused any complications. When the needle is then withdrawn, liquid vitreous will sometimes escape through the needle tract into the subconjunctival space. This is a fortuitous development which will probably eliminate the need for paracentesis. Vitreous incarceration in the pars plana injection site probably occurs but is not known to cause clinically significant complications. Escape of gas into the subconjunctival space is not harmful but may not leave enough gas in the vitreous cavity.

As an alternative to rotating the head prior to withdrawing the needle, a cotton-tipped applicator can be used to occlude the perforation site. The gas escapes instantly upon removal of the needle, so the applicator must be pressed against the shaft of the needle and rolled immediately over the hole as the needle is withdrawn. The head is then rotated 90°.

After gas injection

Following injection, the eye is then examined with the indirect ophthalmoscope to make the following three determinations:

1. *Is the central retinal artery occluded?* Occlusion of the central retinal artery can be safely observed for 10 minutes (Hilton 1986). During this time, the intraocular pressure declines and the artery may reopen. If more than 0.5 ml was injected without egress of liquid vitreous, paracentesis will usually be needed and one can proceed directly to this step. If the artery has not reopened within 10 minutes, paracentesis should be performed (see 'Special procedures').

2. *Is a single gas bubble present or are there multiple small bubbles ('fish eggs')?* Fish eggs are undesirable because a small gas bubble can get through a retinal break into the subretinal space. See 'Special procedures' below for suggestions on management of fish eggs.

3. *Is the bubble mobile within the vitreous or is it trapped at the injection site?* If the bubble is beneath the pars plana epithelium or

trapped in the space bordered by the pars plana, the anterior hyaloid face, and the lens (the canal of Petit), it will not move when the head is turned and will take on a semicircular shape. This has been termed the 'doughnut sign', the 'sausage sign' or the 'bagel sign'. Management of this rare occurrence is discussed below under 'Special procedures'.

The 'steamroller' technique is now used if indicated (see 'Special procedures'). We instil steroid-antibiotic ointment and patch the eye. The meridian of the retinal break is marked by an arrow on the patch to indicate to the patient and family the head position which is to be maintained. We have a hand-held mirror available to show the patient that the head should be positioned so that the arrow is pointing directly at the ceiling. The patient is discharged home and seen for follow-up the next day.

SPECIAL PROCEDURES

Paracentesis

The intended paracentesis site should be resterilized with Betadine solution unless strict sterility has been maintained. A 30-gauge $\frac{1}{2}$-inch needle on a 1-ml syringe with the plunger removed is passed obliquely into the anterior chamber through the limbus, staying over the iris with the bevel up. Fluid will flow passively into the syringe. As the chamber shallows, gentle pressure on the central cornea with a cotton-tipped applicator will deepen the peripheral angle and facilitate fluid egress (Fig. 9.2). Usually no more than 0.2 ml needs to be removed.

If the posterior lens capsule is absent or open, paracentesis should not be performed through the limbus, to avoid incarceration of vitreous in the limbal needle tract. Pass the needle through the pars plana, then angle it into the anterior chamber.

Re-examine the central retinal artery to ensure its patency. As long as the central artery is open (widely patent or with strong pulsation), measurement of the intraocular pressure has little meaning. The pressure will soon return to normal and not increase, even though the gas is expanding (Hilton & Grizzard 1986).

If there has been recent cataract surgery (within six weeks), it is recommended to perform paracentesis before gas injection. If the amount of aqueous removed is less than the planned volume of gas, one should also aspirate liquid vitreous. This will prevent dehiscence of the cataract wound. Cryopexy will also stress the unhealed wound; therefore, laser is recommended.

Fish eggs

'Fish eggs' are usually due to faulty injection technique. In probable order of importance, the following steps will usually prevent this occurrence:

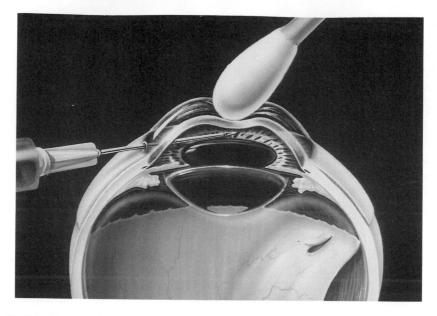

Fig. 9.2   Paracentesis. To perform paracentesis, use a 30-gauge $\frac{1}{2}$-inch needle on a 1-ml syringe with the plunger removed. Pass the needle obliquely through the limbus into the anterior chamber, keeping the needle tip bevel up over the iris. By gently indenting the central cornea with a cotton-tipped applicator, the peripheral chamber deepens at the needle tip, allowing removal of more fluid.

1. Make sure that the needle is shallowly within the vitreous at the time of injection
2. Make sure that the injection site is uppermost
3. Inject with the needle vertical
4. Inject briskly but not too briskly.

If fish eggs do occur, they can usually be caused to coalesce by flicking the eye with a cotton-tipped applicator or finger. Turn the eye so that sclera without underlying retinal breaks is uppermost and flick this site moderately firmly. If this does not cause the bubbles to coalesce, the patient should stay strictly positioned to keep the bubbles away from retinal breaks. If all retinal breaks are tiny, this may not be necessary, but keep in mind that breaks can stretch a little. The bubbles will usually coalesce spontaneously within 24 hours, and then the patient can adopt a position with the retinal break uppermost.

Gas entrapment at the injection site

Following gas injection, if the gas bubble remains trapped at the injection site, it is trapped in the canal of Petit or possibly beneath the pars plana epithelium. If the trapped bubble is small, no treatment is necessary. A large trapped bubble can be removed by passing a 25- or 27-gauge needle back through the injection site. This needle is mounted on a syringe with a small amount of sterile saline, with the plunger removed. The injection site is positioned uppermost and the needle is passed vertically into the bubble. Sometimes it takes a little manipulating to break the surface tension of the bubble and get it to escape. Most of the gas will escape, bubbling up through the fluid in the syringe. At another site, reinject the gas deeper into the vitreous, with 4–5 mm of the needle in the globe.

If macular attachment is not threatened, face-down positioning is a good alternative. We have seen trapped anterior gas bubbles break through the anterior hyaloid face by their own buoyancy, aided by their expansion.

Steamroller

If bullous subretinal fluid extends almost to the macula, placement of a bubble against the bullous detachment may cause macular detachment (Yeo et al 1986). This complication can be easily avoided by the 'steamroller' technique (Hilton et al 1987).

Following injection of the gas bubble, the patient's head is turned to a face-down position in such a way as to cause the bubble to traverse attached retina en route to the macula. Over 5–15 minutes, the patient's head position is very gradually changed until the retinal break is uppermost, causing the bubble to roll toward the retinal break, pushing the subretinal fluid back into the vitreous and flattening the retina (Fig. 9.3).

Subretinal fluid will be expressed through the retinal break into the vitreous cavity at a rate depending on the size of the break. Since cryopexy causes liberation of pigment epithelial cells, which may cause proliferative vitreoretinopathy if they get in the vitreous cavity, cryopexy should not be performed prior to steamrolling.

Whether steamrolling is necessary to prevent macular detachment depends on several factors:

1. How close the detachment is to the macula; only detachments well within the arcades usually need steamrolling
2. How bullous the detachment is
3. How large the gas bubble is.

Possible indications for steamrolling are as follows:

1. Prevention of iatrogenic macular detachment
2. Prevention of iatrogenic detachment of an attached retinal break
3. Reduction of a bullous detachment overhanging the optic nerve, preventing visualization of the central retinal artery during the procedure
4. Reduction of subretinal fluid to encourage more rapid resolution of retinal detachment. This might be of use in cases where all retinal breaks cannot be covered at one time by the gas bubble.

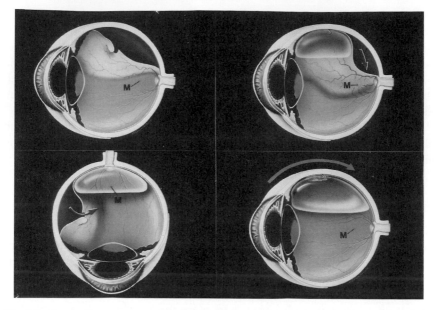

Fig. 9.3 Steamroller manoeuvre. Top left: bullous retinal detachment threatens to detach the macula. Top right: placement of a gas bubble against the peripheral detachment may cause extension of the detachment into the macula (arrow). Bottom left: to prevent macular detachment, the 'steamroller' technique is used. The gas bubble is injected away from the area of detachment and the patient's head is positioned to manoeuvre the gas bubble into the macula without passing through detached retina. Subretinal fluid starts to escape from the subretinal space into the vitreous cavity (arrow) as the bubble impinges on the detachment. Bottom right: over 5–15 minutes, the patient's head is gradually rotated to make the retinal break uppermost (arrow). This may be repeated if necessary. Subretinal fluid has thus been pushed away from the macula, preventing macular detachment. Reproduced with permission from J. B. Lippinott Company, Journal of Ophthalmology.

POSTOPERATIVE MANAGEMENT

Plain acetaminophen (Tylenol) is usually sufficient for postoperative pain control. We recommend considerable restriction in activity initially, liberalizing day by day as the retina reattaches, the chorioretinal scar matures, and finally the gas bubble resorbs. The patient is allowed to return to work two weeks after the procedure. He should be advised not to fly until the bubble is gone or is quite small.

If all retinal breaks are closed, the subretinal fluid usually resorbs within 24–48 hours. If the fluid is not resorbing, a break has been overlooked or the patient has not been positioned properly.

Ensuring proper patient positioning requires considerable effort. It is helpful to explain to the patient why positioning is important and to demonstrate the position which allows the bubble to close the breaks. The neck strain of an oblique head position can be eased by explaining that standing with the head tilted 45° to the left is the same as lying on a couch with the head tilted 45° to the right.

Patient positioning is maintained during waking hours for five days; however, three days is probably adequate. The patient should not sleep face up, to avoid gas-induced cataract formation in the phakic eye, or ciliary-block glaucoma in the aphakic eye.

We see the patient on the first postoperative day. Depending on resolution of subretinal fluid, the next follow-up is in two days, then four days later, then one week, two weeks, one, two, and four months later. The purpose of this frequent schedule is largely to look for new retinal breaks. These breaks do not tend to jeopardize the outcome if close follow-up results in early detection and treatment (Tornambe et al 1989).

Inferior subretinal fluid sometimes persists for weeks or months. As long as the fluid is not increasing and the macula is attached, reoperation is not necessary.

INDICATIONS

The inclusion criteria for the multicentre clinical trial excluded cases with the following characteristics:

1. Breaks larger than one clock hour or multiple breaks extending over more than one clock hour of the retina
2. Breaks in the inferior four clock hours of the retina
3. Presence of proliferative vitreoretinopathy grade C or D (Retina Society Terminology Committee 1983)
4. Physical disability or mental incompetence precluding maintenance of the required positioning
5. Severe or uncontrolled glaucoma
6. Cloudy media precluding full assessment of the retina.

Subsequent experience has demonstrated that selected cases that do not strictly meet these criteria can be successfully treated with pneumatic retinopexy (Tornambe et al 1988).

Extent of breaks

Clearly, breaks spanning more than one clock hour can be treated with penumatic retinopexy. Single or multiple tears spanning three clock hours pose no particular problem. Detached tears six clock hours apart are difficult to fix with pneumatic retinopexy, although alternating positioning can be used. Even detachments with giant retinal tears have been cured with pneumatic retinopexy (Lahey & Irvine 1990). The size of the gas bubble should reflect the size of the problem.

When deciding whether a case is amenable to pneumatic retinopexy, recognize that there is a difference between attached and detached breaks. In cases where an attached break is present on the opposite side of the eye from the detached breaks, alternate positioning would not be needed. The attached break should probably be treated with laser prior to the gas injection. Care should then be taken, such as by using the steamroller technique, to prevent the bubble from pushing the subretinal fluid into the attached break and causing it to detach. By following these two steps, multiple dispersed attached breaks may be ignored in positioning and calculation of bubble size.

Inferior breaks

Most cases with breaks in the inferior four clock hours of the eye have been difficult to treat with pneumatic retinopexy, in spite of various attempts (Tornambe et al 1988). Even for supple patients, it is very difficult to tilt the head below the horizontal for very long. In our opinion, a detached break in the inferior four clock hours represents a contraindication to pneumatic retinopexy. The difference between attached and detached breaks should again be recognized. Attached inferior breaks do not necessarily contraindicate pneumatic retinopexy if treated with laser and steamrolling as described above.

Proliferative vitreoretinopathy (PVR)

Since pneumatic retinopexy does not relieve traction like scleral buckling or vitrectomy does, significant preoperative traction on a retinal tear is a relative contraindication to the pneumatic procedure. When a tear is adjacent to a star fold, pneumatic retinopexy is probably not the procedure of choice. Mild to moderate proliferative vitreoretinopathy which is distant from any retinal breaks generally does not contraindicate pneumatic retinopexy. More severe PVR requires scleral buckling or vitrectomy.

Inability to maintain positioning

Failure to maintain faithfully the appropriate position is probably an important cause of failure of pneumatic retinopexy. It is important to inquire regarding back or neck problems and to assess mental competence before deciding on pneumatic retinopexy. Recognize that some positions are quite easy to maintain while others require excellent cooperation. Positioning is easiest with tears between 11 and 1 o'clock.

Glaucoma

Glaucoma has proved to be relatively unimportant as a contraindication to pneumatic retinopexy. The large majority of glaucoma patients can be treated with pneumatic retinopexy without problem. Patients with quite severe glaucoma, such as with splitting of the macular field due to glaucoma, might suffer noticeable damage even from brief elevations in intraocular pressure, and pneumatic retinopexy might be contraindicated. Except in cases of severely impaired trabecular outflow facility, serial measurements of intraocular pressure following gas injection is not necessary.

Cloudy media

It is important to the success of pneumatic retinopexy that all retinal breaks be identified and treated. Opacities such as peripheral vitreous haemorrhage represent relative contraindications to pneumatic retinopexy. Since pneumatic retinopexy does not seem to jeopardize an eye for future scleral buckling if needed, it may not be unreasonable to use the pneumatic procedure even when opacities obscure part of the attached retina, but this represents a calculated risk.

Several other conditions warrant comment as potential relative contraindications.

Lattice degeneration

In several series, patients with extensive lattice degeneration tended to do rather poorly with pneumatic retinopexy. It does not appear that mild to moderate lattice should be considered a contraindication.

Aphakia/pseudophakia

In some series, aphakic eyes did poorly with pneumatic retinopexy, but in other reports this was not the case. Aphakic eyes, prone to multiple tiny far-peripheral holes, require an especially careful preoperative examination. With peripheral capsular opacities frequently present, the view of the peripheral retina can be quite limited. Such cases should probably not be done with pneumatic retinopexy. In our opinion, if the peripheral retina can be adequately examined, aphakia or pseudophakia is not a contraindication to pneumatic retinopexy. Experience has shown that eyes with an open posterior capsule tend to do less well than eyes with the capsule intact (McAllister et al 1988). Like severe lattice degeneration, aphakia/pseudophakia with an open posterior capsule warrants extra caution.

Pneumatic retinopexy has particular advantages in the management of several types of cases.

Macular holes and other posterior retinal breaks

Posterior retinal breaks are difficult to treat with scleral buckling. Pneumatic retinopexy is the procedure of choice in many of these cases. It has also been reported as an option in the treatment of optic pits with serous macular detachment (Flynn 1989).

Redetachment following scleral buckling

When subretinal fluid accumulates due to a superior break following scleral buckling, pneumatic retinopexy may be much easier than revising the buckle.

Isolated tears under the superior rectus

Placing a segmental buckle under a vertically acting muscle runs the risk of iatrogenic diplopia, eliminated with pneumatic retinopexy.

Contraindications to general anaesthesia

Since most scleral buckling is done under a general anaesthetic, medical contraindications to general anaesthesia may indicate pneumatic retinopexy.

COMPLICATIONS

Subretinal gas

We are unaware of any reported cases of subretinal gas in the absence of fish eggs at the time of injection. If fish eggs are noted following injection, one should examine carefully for the presence of subretinal gas. Once the gas bubble expands it may be more difficult to get it back out of the break it passed through. In none of the cases in the series of McDonald et al (1987) was the subretinal gas noted immediately after injection. If a gas bubble does get beneath the retina, it gives the detached retina a pearly, dome-shaped, refractive sheen (Fig. 9.4).

Attempt first to massage the bubble back toward the retinal break by scleral depression assisted by positioning as needed. If this fails and the amount of

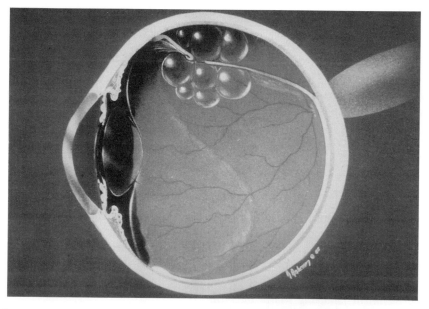

Fig. 9.4 Subretinal gas. When 'fish eggs' (multiple small gas bubbles) occur, several bubbles may pass through the retinal break into the subretinal space. By courtesy of R G Chenowith, Oregon

subretinal gas is large, prompt surgical removal with vitrectomy is probably required. Smaller bubbles can be managed conservatively. In spite of the subretinal bubble, the break can usually be secluded from liquid vitreous with strict positioning, and subretinal fluid will resorb. The smaller subretinal bubble will resorb before the larger vitreous bubble and the detachment can be repaired, injecting additional gas if needed.

Iatrogenic macular detachment

This preventable complication is avoided by using the steamroller technique as described above.

New retinal breaks

New or missed retinal breaks following pneumatic retinopexy occurred in 13% of 1274 eyes (Hilton 1990). This high incidence mandates close postoperative follow-up. In the multicentre trial, 96% of eyes with new breaks were successfully reattached (Tornambe et al 1989). Approximately half of such breaks were managed in the outpatient department without scleral buckling. New breaks can often be treated easily with pneumatic techniques, without automatically resorting to scleral buckling.

PVR

Pneumatic retinopexy does not appear to increase the incidence of PVR. In the multicentre clinical trial, PVR occurred in 5% of eyes following scleral buckling and 3% of eyes following pneumatic retinopexy (Tornambe et al 1989). It may be possible to reduce the incidence of PVR by replacing cryopexy of detached breaks with laser treatment of reattached breaks.

COMPARISON WITH SCLERAL BUCKLING

A multicentre, controlled, randomized clinical trial with 198 patients compared pneumatic retinopexy with scleral buckling (Tornambe et al 1989). The key findings of this study are shown in Table 9.2.

Comparison of the two procedures is summarized as follows:

1.   Postoperative visual acuity is significantly better with pneumatic retinopexy than with scleral buckling for eyes where the macula was detached for less than 14 days ($P = 0.01$).
2.   Anatomical results are not significantly different.
3.   Complications are similar, based on a score system which weighted heavily the need for postoperative laser or cryo.
4.   Morbidity is less with pneumatic retinopexy.
5.   Cost is generally much less with pneumatic retinopexy.

Table 9.2   Summary of findings of the multicentre randomized controlled clinical trial (Tornambe et al 1989)

Results of randomized controlled clinical trial	Scleral buckling	Pneumatic retinopexy	P value
Anatomical success			
With one operation ± laser or cryo	84%	81%	NS
Final reattachment	98%	99%	NS
Visual results[a]			
20/50 or better	56%	80%	0.01
Worse than 20/50	43%	20%	NC
Morbidity[b]	Moderate	Mild	0.001
Complications			
New/missed breaks	13%	23%	0.05
Choroidal detachment	17%	3%	0.001
Myopic shift	68%	3%	0.001
PVR	5%	3%	NS

[a] At six months in eyes with preoperative macular detachment for 14 days or less. Visual acuity was also significantly better for pneumatic retinopexy than for scleral buckling when all eyes were compared ($P = 0.01$).
[b] 'Morbidity' includes severity and duration of the following parameters: pain, diplopia, nausea, strabismus, pseudoptosis, and conjunctival haemorrhage ($P = 0.001$ for most parameters).
NS = not significant; NC = not calculated.

    6.   Scleral buckling is the more versatile procedure, with some detachments not amenable to pneumatic retinopexy. At least 40% of detachments are candidates for pneumatic retinopexy. However, pneumatic retinopexy can treat some detachments which scleral buckling cannot, such as detachments with very posterior breaks.
    7.   The main disadvantage of pneumatic retinopexy is the need for postoperative positioning and close follow-up care.

Pneumatic retinopexy is more versatile than the temporary episcleral balloon, being able to treat larger breaks, more widely spread breaks, and more posterior breaks than the balloon can treat. However, the balloon can treat detached inferior breaks which the bubble cannot.

KEY POINTS TO CLINICAL PRACTICE

Pneumatic retinopexy is a new outpatient procedure for the repair of selected retinal detachments. No surgical incisions are required. A gas bubble is injected into the vitreous cavity, and laser or cryopexy is applied. The anatomical success rate is comparable to scleral buckling, but the morbidity is less and the visual results are significantly better with pneumatic retinopexy than with scleral buckling. It should be considered in cases without inferior or extensive retinal breaks or severe PVR.

REFERENCES

Campochiaro P A, Kaden I H, Vidaurri-Leal J, Glaser B M 1985 Cryotherapy enhances intravitreal dispersion of viable retinal pigment epithelial cells. Arch Ophthalmol 103: 434–436

Escoffery R F, Olk R J, Grand M G, Boniuk I 1985 Vitrectomy without scleral buckling for primary rhegmatogenous retinal detachment. Am J Ophthalmol 99: 275–281

Flynn H W 1989 Treatment options for optic pits, presented at the Second International Conference on Pneumatic Retinopexy, Tampa, Florida, October 6

Friberg T R 1989 Laser photocoagulation to produce chorioretinal adhesion, presented at the Second International Conference on Pneumatic Retinopexy, Tampa, Florida, October 6

Friberg T R, Eller A W 1988 Pneumatic repair of primary and secondary retinal detachments using a binocular indirect ophthalmoscope laser delivery system. Ophthalmology 95: 187–193

Griffith R D, Ryan E A, Hilton G F 1976 Primary retinal detachments without apparent breaks. Am J Ophthalmol 81: 420–427

Hilton G F 1986 Planned elevation of intraocular pressure with temporary closure of the central retinal artery during retinal surgery. Arch Ophthalmol 104: 975

Hilton G F, Tornambe P E, Brinton D et al 1990 The complications of pneumatic retinopexy. Trans Am Ophthalmol Soc 88: 191–210

Hilton G F, Grizzard W S 1986 Pneumatic retinopexy: a two-step outpatient operation without conjunctival incision. Ophthalmology 93: 626–640

Hilton G F, Kelly N E, Salzano T C et al 1987 Pneumatic retinopexy: a collaborative report of the first 100 cases. Ophthalmology 94: 307–314

Humayun M S, Yeo J H, Koski W S, Michels R G 1989 The rate of sulfur hexafluoride escape from a plastic syringe. Arch Ophthalmol 107: 853–854

Lahey J M, Irvine A R 1990 A case of giant retinal tear repaired by pneumatic retinopexy. Presented at the Cordes Eye Society Meeting, San Francisco, California, April 5

McAllister I L, Fraco, Meyers S M et al 1988 Comparison of pneumatic retinopexy with alternative surgical techniques. Ophthalmology 95: 877–883

McDonald H R, Abrams G W, Irvine A R et al 1987 The management of subretinal gas following attempted pneumatic retinal reattachment. Ophthalmology 94: 319–326

Norton E W D 1973 Intraocular gas in the management of selected retinal detachments. Trans Am Acad Ophthalmol Otolaryngol 77: OP85–98

Ohm J 1911 Uber die Behandlung der Netzhautablosung durch operative Entleerung der subretinalen Flussigkeit und Einspritzung von Luft in den Glaskorper. Graefes Arch Clin Exp Ophthalmol 79: 442–450

Packo K H 1989 Gas injection techniques, presented at the Second International Conference on Pneumatic Retinopexy, Tampa, Florida, October 6

Parver L M, Lincoff H 1977 Geometry of intraocular gas used in retinal surgery. Mod Probl Ophthalmol 18: 338–343

Retina Society Terminology Committee 1983 The classification of retinal detachment with proliferative vitreoretinopathy. Ophthalmology 90: 121–125

Schaffer R N 1985 Presented in discussion at the American Ophthalmological Society, Hot Springs, Virginia, March 19–22

Tornambe P E, Hilton G F, Kelly N F et al 1988 Expanded indications for pneumatic retinopexy. Ophthalmology 95: 597–600

Tornambe P E, Hilton G F, Retinal Detachment Study Group 1989 Pneumatic retinopexy: a multicentre randomized controlled clinical trial comparing pneumatic retinopexy with scleral buckling. Ophthalmology 96: 772–784

Yeo J H, Vidaurri-Leal J, Glaser B M 1986 Extension of retinal detachments as a complication of pneumatic retinopexy. Arch Ophthalmol 104: 1161–1163

10

Charged particle irradiation of melanoma of the choroid

D. H. Char   J. R. Castro

INTRODUCTION

While ionizing radiation has been used to treat uveal melanomas since 1929, a number of issues remain unresolved (Moore 1930, Char et al 1989b). In this review we have tried to summarize our understanding of the data on charged particle (helium ion and proton) radiation of uveal melanoma, and to point out areas that require further elucidation.

Initial attempts to use radiation to destroy uveal melanoma and retain the globe were performed with radon seeds (no longer used because of their public health hazard), and cobalt and ruthenium brachytherapy (radioactive plaques). Ruthenium has limited applicability since it is a beta-emitting isotope that had very short-range tissue penetration, hence can only be used for relatively thin tumours (Lommatzsch 1983, Busse et al 1983). Most early experience utilized ^{60}Co radioactive plaques (Stallard 1959, 1961, 1968). A number of clinicians observed complications of treatment (Stallard 1933, MacFaul & Bedford 1970, Bedford et al 1970, Char et al 1977). Radiation vascular damage with resultant visual loss was frequent. Complications of treatment were felt to be mainly due to diffuse ocular radiation delivered because ^{60}Co is a very penetrant source of gamma radiation. In Stallard's experience, only 40% of irradiated eyes that were retained had a final visual acuity of 6/18 or better (MacFaul 1977). Similarly, a review of a larger cobalt brachytherapy experience in Philadelphia showed that less than 50% of treated patients retained 'useful vision' five years after treatment (Brady et al 1988).

Charged particle irradiation using either protons or helium ions was initiated in two centres in the USA in the late 1970s (Gragoudas et al 1977, Char et al 1980). The first clinical experience with these types of radiation therapy was initiated at our institution for treatment of pituitary disease in 1954 (Tobias 1985, Boone et al 1977). Animal experiments with proton beam irradiation of simulated eye masses were published in 1975 (Constable et al 1975).

There were three theoretical reasons to consider either helium ions or proton radiation to treat uveal melanomas. First, because of the inherent Bragg peak with charged particle irradiation, it is much more focusable than any form of brachytherapy; with helium ions the lateral and distal spread of

169

radiation decreases from 100% of dose to less than 10% of dose in approximately 1.5 mm. Second, unlike radioactive plaques that have an inherent radiation dose gradient between the scleral surface and the tumour apex, uniform dosage is delivered to the entire tumour with both protons and helium ions. We believed, and the data have generally borne us out, that the absence of a dose gradient might allow larger tumours to be treated than possible with any form of brachytherapy. Third, it was initially thought that uveal melanomas were relatively radiation-resistant tumours; at the cellular level, linear energy transfer (LET) associated with helium and heavier particles is often more effective against radio-resistant neoplasms (Tobias 1985). A number of other features of charged particle irradiation are attractive for uveal melanoma therapy. There is no radiation exposure to medical personnel. Only a single surgical procedure is necessary to localize the tumour for particles; brachytherapy requires both plaque insertion and removal. There would be a significantly lower incidence of secondary strabismus after placement of tantalum marker rings, especially in tumours that were partially under an extraocular muscle. In such locations, often either the radioactive plaque stretches the overlying muscle, or the muscle has to be disinserted to treat the scleral tumour surface with the brachytherapy source.

CHARGED PARTICLE TREATMENT TECHNIQUE

After the diagnosis of uveal melanoma is made, and informed consent for charged particle therapy is obtained, patients are taken to the operating room, and the scleral surface of the tumour is localized with both diffuse corneal transillumination as well as indirect ophthalmoscopy with point source transillumination. The tumour margins are delineated by suturing four 2.5-mm tantalum marker rings on the scleral circumference of the uveal melanoma. A computer program is used to develop an optimal treatment plan that incorporates surgical data, fundus drawing, standardized A-scan and wide angle fundus photographs (Goitein & Miller 1983). The goal of treatment planning is to encompass the tumour plus a 2.5-mm surround of presumably normal choroid (to avoid a marginal miss) in the high-dose region, while avoiding, as much as possible, radiation of the fovea, optic nerve, lens and cornea. After a sufficient postoperative recovery period, so that the patient can both tolerate an eyelid speculum and move and hold their eye in an appropriate gaze angle, treatment is performed on an outpatient basis. Different head fixation devices have been used to immobilize the patient, and orthogonal X-ray is used to localize the tumour for each treatment. In Boston, Switzerland and San Francisco patients are simulated, then treated in either four or five fractions in seven to ten days. Radiation dosages used for protons or helium ions have varied from 50 to 100 gray equivalents (GyE). The relative biological effect of charged particles is not the same as with conventional photon radiation beams; gray equivalents equal physical gray multiplied by relative biological effect (1.1 for protons and 1.3 for helium ions) (Blakely et al 1985).

CHARGED PARTICLE TREATMENT DATA

Approximately 2000 patients have been treated with charged particles in Boston, San Francisco, Villigen (Switzerland), Japan, Clatterbridge (UK) and Moscow (Gragoudas et al 1977, Char et al 1980, Char et al 1990, Egan et al 1989, Gragoudas et al 1987, Chuvilo et al 1984, Brovkina & Zarubei 1986, Zografos et al 1988). In the first three centres similar localization and treatment techniques have been used. Most of the Russian data are on smaller anterior uveal melanomas using different localization and treatment techniques; their criteria for treatment efficacy is difficult to evaluate (Chuvilo et al 1984, Brovkina & Zarubei 1986). The longest follow-up data are available from Boston and San Francisco and it is concordant. The following data are reviewed from these two American centres.

Most patients have had large uveal melanomas; <10% of patients treated at either institution have had small tumours, defined as less than 10 mm in diameter and less than 3 mm thick. Approximately 65% of patients we have treated have tumours >15 mm in diameter and/or >5 mm thick. The mean uveal melanoma thickness treated with helium ions was 6.1 mm (Char et al 1990). In both centres approximately 90% of treated eyes were retained five years after radiation, and the five-year tumour-related mortality was between 18% and 20% (Char et al 1990, Gragoudas et al 1988).

Prognostic factors in irradiated patients are similar to those observed in patients treated with enucleation (Char et al 1990, Gragoudas et al 1988). Poorer prognosis after charged particle irradiation is a function of increased patient age, largest tumour diameter, location of the anterior edge of the melanoma vis à vis the equator and ciliary body, and the presence of extrascleral extension. In our experience, <10% of patients with tumours <16 mm in diameter and <8 mm thick developed widespread disease; most metastases occurred in patients with larger tumours. Approximately one-third of patients with a largest tumour diameter greater than 15 mm developed metastatic disease (Char et al 1990). In the Boston experience, the mean interval between treatment and the detection of metastatic disease was 2.1 years (range 3 months to 7.5 years; in San Francisco the mean interval was 39 months) (Char et al 1990, Gragoudas et al 1988).

It is difficult to compare survival rates after different forms of therapy since selection criteria used to choose a type of treatment usually has important prognostic ramifications. In a retrospective study, Seddon et al (1985) compared survival of proton-irradiated patients with matched, enucleated patients managed by other New England ophthalmologists. Using appropriate statistical analysis, survival after charged particle irradiation was better ($\chi^2 = 6.47$, $p < 0.01$). In other studies comparing survival after brachytherapy or enucleation, no significant difference was noted (Char 1989a).

There has been a major change in our understanding of tumour radiation effect since the early studies of ocular radiation for uveal melanoma. Initially most investigators assumed that if the tumour was not completely obliterated it was still active. Some investigators still have this misconception, even though modern radiobiology has shown that the major goal of radiation is to destroy the reproductive integrity of a neoplasm (Lawton 1989, Manschot & Van Strik 1987, Suit & Gallagher 1964, Tolmach 1961). It is uncertain why, but the eye is a relatively inefficient site for removal of tumour debris. We and others have noted that some tumours that became almost entirely necrotic did not demonstrate significant shrinkage after therapy (Goodman et al 1986, Oosterhuis et al 1988, Bujara & Hallerman 1984). Less than 10% of uveal melanomas treated with proton irradiation are reduced to flat scars (Gragoudas et al 1987). In our experience with eyes that have been removed because of late radiation complications, but had no evidence of either recurrent or continued tumour growth, reproductive integrity has been destroyed as detected by two different types of assays. In these enucleated eyes, no evidence of tumour cell mitoses were noted on standard light microscopy (Crawford & Char 1987). In addition, most of those patients received intravenous bromodeoxyuridine, a thymidine analogue, prior to enucleation. This agent is only taken up by cells that are actively cycling, and none of these irradiated melanomas showed evidence of active DNA synthesis (Char et al 1989a).

Patterns of ocular tumour response to treatment are correlated with tumour-related mortality. An early, rapid tumour regression is associated with a poorer prognosis for life after either charged particle or radioactive plaque therapy (Augsburger et al 1987, Glynn et al 1989). Probably this occurs because more malignant tumours grow rapidly and have a higher percentage of cycling cells. The major effect of radiation is when cells enter mitosis, and a rapidly dividing uveal melanoma would therefore both grow and shrink more rapidly than a less aggressive tumour.

After either brachytherapy or charged particle radiation, detectable tumour response is delayed. Five charges are usually noted at different intervals after therapy: loss of an exudative retinal detachment; decreased tumour thickness; change in the tumour's coloration to a dull, charcoal grey; loss of homogeneity on ultrasonography; and loss of vascularity on fluorescein angiography. Usually the first detectable post-treatment response is loss of subretinal fluid; it has a mean latency of six months. Over 90% of successfully treated uveal melanomas have documented tumour shrinkage; in 10% of cases no shrinkage is noted although some of these melanomas may be entirely necrotic (Goodman et al 1986). Usually shrinkage can be detected either clinically or on ultrasound examination between three and 18 months (mean one year) after either helium ion or proton irradiation. The mean tumour shrinkage is approximately 40% (Char et al 1989b). As would be expected, patients who are treated with charged particle radiation and have recurrent or continued intraocular tumour growth do less well than those whose tumours are controlled (Char et al 1990).

A number of complications have been observed after ocular radiation, even with highly focused charged particle beams. Some of the eye damage observed can be explained on the basis of a direct radiation effect, while other components cannot. In our experience, approximately 50% of uveal melanomas examined in our ocular oncology unit have the posterior tumour edge within 3 mm of the optic nerve and/or fovea (Char 1984). Unfortunately, in order to treat a tumour in this location, with an adequate margin to avoid incomplete coverage, sufficient radiation is delivered to visually vital structures usually to decrease vision over a five-year interval. Anterior segment damage also occurs as a direct result of the entrance beam (Char et al 1980). The Bragg peak is expanded so that the entire tumour volume is included in the high-dose treatment field; as a result the radiation dose in the eye anterior to the Bragg peak is at approximately 70% of maximum. This entrance dose is responsible for the eyelash loss, conjunctival telangiectasia, and much of the neovascular glaucoma and cataract that has occurred after particle irradiation. Neovascular glaucoma occurs in approximately 10% of charged particle treated patients; it is most common in larger, anterior uveal melanomas (Kim et al 1986). In a series reported by Egan et al (1989) neovascular glaucoma accounted for almost 50% of enucleations after proton beam irradiation. In our experience with a randomized, prospective dynamically balanced trial comparing ^{125}I brachytherapy with helium ion irradiation, neovascular glaucoma is statistically significantly more common after charged particle as compared with radioactive plaque therapy (Char 1989b) Other direct radiation complications observed include in field vasculopathy (cotton wool spots, microaneurysms, vessel closure, hard exudates), cystoid macular oedema and optic neuropathy (Stallard 1933, MacFaul & Bedford 1970, Bedford et al 1970). As Stallard first described in 1933, direct radiation vascular damage to the retina can produce the above findings and resultant visual loss. The mean latency of detection of these complications after cobalt plaques is between two and three years; visual loss from radiation vasculopathy after charged particles occurs somewhat more rapidly (mean 18 months) (Char et al 1977, Char et al 1980, Linstadt et al 1988).

Some complications are multifactorial. As an example, almost 15% of eyes treated by enucleation alone for large, uveal melanomas had rubeosis (Cappin 1973). Similarly, we have examined patients prior to radiation with retinal neovascularization, optic disc neovascularization, vessel closure, exudates and cystoid macular oedema. Probably cytokines produced by both the tumour and the host inflammatory/immunological cells contribute to ocular morbidity (Char 1989b). In both the Boston and San Francisco experience, increased tumour thickness, independent of location vis à vis the optic nerve and fovea, is a poor prognostic indicator for both vision and loss of the eye. Figure 10.1 and 2 shows an 8.5-mm thick peripheral uveal tumour treated with helium ion irradiation, with good tumour control. Treatment planning and other studies confirmed that essentially no radiation was delivered to the posterior pole, yet one and a half years later visual acuity was diminished because of

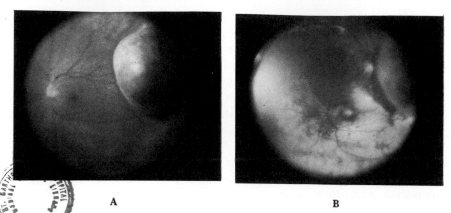

A   B

Fig. 10.1 A Large peripheral melanoma prior to treatment with helium ion irradiation. No radiation was delivered posterior to the equator. Good tumour resolution occurred. (Reprinted from Char 1989a.) B Clinical photograph of the posterior pole of tumour shown in Figure 3.1, one year later. At the time of initial treatment vision was 20/20. One year later, despite no radiation to the posterior pole, visually destructive maculopathy developed. The absence of radiation in this area is consistent with the hypothesis that other factors including intrinsic tumour cytokines and lymphokines are important in post-treatment ocular morbidity. (Reprinted from Char 1989a.)

macular exudation. This case is a good illustration of ocular morbidity that occurred not directly due to radiation. Inflammation and intrinsic tumour factors probably produced the major component of ocular damage in this case. The observation that some post-radiation neovascular glaucomas can be controlled with topical corticosteroid drops alone is consistent with the concept that inflammatory cells and their products are also important in the induction of radiation complications. As discussed below, multivariate aetiology of ocular morbidity is an important concept, since some attempts to diminish visual loss after radiation are mainly predicated on lowering radiation dose. While these may decrease direct radiation toxicity, it is doubtful they will alleviate damage due to these other causes.

Overall, a combination of patient age, tumour factors (thickness, location and diameter) and both radiation effects and host/tumour response to therapy affect the ultimate visual outcome. In the combined experience in San Francisco and Boston, approximately 40% of patients who have an initial visual acuity of 6/12 or better retain it four years after treatment (Char et al 1990, Char 1984, Linstadt et al 1988). Overall, approximately one-third of patients have a final visual acuity of 6/12 or better after charged particle therapy. While these long-term visual results appear to mirror those reported by Stallard, it must be kept in mind that the size and location of tumours treated with cobalt plaques as compared with modern charged particle beams are quite disparate. Most of Stallard's cases were small or medium-sized melanomas, while most treated with particles have been either large or very large. Proximity to the nerve and fovea, maximum tumour thickness, pretreatment vision, pretreatment exudative retinal detachment, and predicted radiation dose to the optic nerve or fovea were important pretreatment indicators for visual loss.

Enucleation was performed in approximately 10–15% of charged particle beam-treated patients within five years of therapy (Char et al 1990, Egan et al 1989). Most eyes were enucleated because of radiation complications, with intractable neovascular glaucoma being the leading cause for eye loss. Less than 4% of treated eyes required enucleation because of either continued tumour growth or regrowth (Char et al 1990, Egan et al 1989). Most local tumour failures occurred early in our experience and were possibly due to suboptimal radiation treatment planning. Rarely a tumour is treated that is more diffuse than is clinically recognized, and this has necessitated either retreatment or enucleation when the untreated portion of the tumour grows and becomes apparent (Crawford & Char 1987). The relatively low incidence of non-technical (i.e. re-simulation showed patient received correct radiation) treatment failures demonstrates that treatment of the tumour with a 2.5-mm surround of normal choroid is sufficient in almost all cases to avoid incomplete coverage of the melanoma. The local failure rate observed with charged particles appears to be less than has been reported with various forms of radioactive plaques where between 10% and 40% of treated eyes were removed because of possible continued or recurrent tumour growth (Stallard 1968, MacFaul 1977, Lommatzsch 1983, Busse et al 1983, Gass 1985, Bosworth et al 1988). The reasons for the disparity in local tumour control between brachytherapy and charged particle are unclear. Probably technical proficiency in radiation oncology and radiation physics, and larger experience with uveal melanomas in ocular oncology centres, partially explain the better results with helium ions and protons. Our prospective randomized study comparing helium ion with ^{125}I brachytherapy should determine if there are other factors that could account for differences in the rates of local tumour control. The stability of radioactive plaques on the scleral surface of the eye may be an important factor. It is possible that the higher failure rate observed in posterior pole melanomas treated with brachytherapy may be due to plaque tilt. This would decrease radiation dose to the posterior portion of the tumour and result in a marginal miss.

A number of questions remain unanswered regarding the use of charged particle radiation in uveal melanoma therapy. While a number of potential advantages of helium ion or proton irradiation have been discussed above, some disadvantages have also become evident.

There are only seven centres in the world where charged particles are currently used to treat uveal melanoma; others are under construction or planned. These units are expensive to build and require sophisticated radiation physics and radiation oncology support staff to provide optimal patient care. The entrance beam of charged particles results in a significantly higher incidence of anterior segment complications as compared with ^{125}I radioactive plaque therapy (Char et al 1989b). As discussed above, in a phase I–II as well as a randomized prospective study, eyelid, conjunctival and corneal complications were more frequent in helium ion-treated patients. In certain ocular locations, especially in the superior temporal or inferior nasal choroid, there is a higher incidence of lacrimal gland or nasolacrimal drainage system damage with particles than when a low-energy gamma source, which can be almost completely shielded with 0.2 mm of gold, such as [125]I (Bosworth et al 1988).

Two major uveal melanoma treatment issues remain unresolved. First, especially in larger treated tumours, there is significant post-treatment morbidity; how can this be decreased? Second, especially in older patients with larger tumours that involve both the choroid and anterior uvea, there is significant tumour-related mortality; how can this be diminished?

As discussed above, there is a multifactorial aetiology for post-treatment complications. Approaches to diminish ocular morbidity include the use of lower radiation doses, using different types of radiation techniques, combining lower radiation with hyperthermia, and resecting tumours.

We retrospectively reviewed the results of a phase I–II radiation dose trial that used 50, 60, 70 or 80 GyE of helium ion irradiation to treat uveal melanomas (Kindy-Degnan et al 1989). The tumour control, enucleation, complications and survival were similar at all dose levels. These data are consistent with the hypothesis that uveal melanomas are not radio-resistant, and significantly less than 100 Gy is needed to control them. Figure 10.2 shows an idealized dose–response curve for uveal melanoma radiation. It is clear that lower radiation doses can be used to control uveal melanomas; however, it is uncertain whether this treatment alteration will diminish non-radiation complications. Unfortunately, even at 50 GyE of helium ion irradiation delivered in five fractions over eight days there is significant

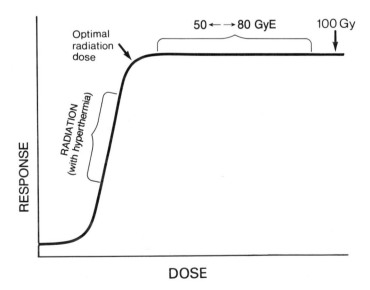

Fig. 10.2   Idealized dose–response curve for uveal melanoma radiation.

radiation vasculopathy. The patient shown in Figure 10.3 had a growing macular melanoma treated with 50 GyE with resultant visual loss several years later. It is likely that other fractionation schedules (much smaller daily doses given over a longer total time) would result in less ocular damage, but other technical, logistic and cost constraints argue against that approach. It is difficult to justify too much dose reduction, since local failure after helium ion irradiation was associated with a poorer prognosis (Char et al 1989b, Glynn et al 1989, Char et al 1990).

A second approach being investigated is to compare different forms of radiation. As discussed above, we have approximately 200 patients in a prospective, dynamically balanced randomized trial comparing helium ion irradiation with ^{125}I brachytherapy (Char et al 1989b). All patients have tumours <15 mm in diameter and <10 mm-thick. The mean follow-up is approximately 30 months; currently there are more anterior segment complications with particles, and more radiation retinopathy with plaques, but visual outcome is still comparable. Further follow-up in these patients will be necessary to determine the relative morbidities associated with these forms of radiation.

A third approach to decrease radiation complications is to combine lower-dose radiation with hyperthermia. In some animal models heat and radiation are both synergistic (or at least additive) and are maximally effective in different phases of the cell cycle (Abe & Hiraoka 1985, Paliwal et al 1989). As an example, hypoxic, acidic cells, or cells in the late synthesis phase of the DNA cell cycle, are relatively radio-resistant but are sensitive to hyperthermia (Abe & Hiraoka 1985, Paliwal et al 1989). A number of different hyperthermia delivery systems are being used to treat experimental models of uveal melanoma, including ultrasound, microwave, conductive heating, ferromagnetic and laser modalities (Coleman et al 1986, Finger et al 1989). There are a number of theoretical and technical problems associated with hyperthermia, and these must be dealt with before this approach can be routinely used in clinical care. It is uncertain how much of an additive effect

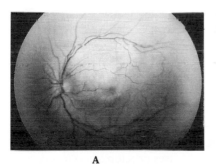
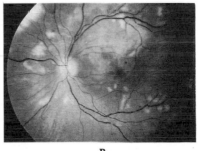

A   B

Fig. 10.3 **A** Growing macular melanoma prior to treatment. **B** Tumour approximately five years after 50 GyE of helium ion irradiation, with good control but visually destructive maculopathy.

hyperthermia has when combined with uveal melanoma radiation. The optimal timing, temperature, monitoring and delivery system for ocular hyperthermia is unknown (Perez et al 1989). In a number of institutions, including our own, human trials have started (Coleman et al 1986, Finger et al 1989). Some clinical data have been reported; however, it must be cautiously interpreted. As an example, Finger et al (1989) have shown tumour control in a small number of patients treated with approximately 70 Gy of brachytherapy and hyperthermia. While these data demonstrate that micro-wave hyperthermia can be delivered to a human uveal melanoma with acceptable morbidity, it does not address its efficacy since with 70 Gy of brachytherapy alone we have maintained over 94% local tumour control. Currently we are starting some prospective trials at much lower radiation doses with hyperthermia; however, it will take at least four years to determine the efficacy of that approach. In addition, there are some obvious theoretical limitations to hyperthermia. It is obvious that some ocular morbidity is a direct result of radiation, and in these cases hyperthermia and a lower radiation dose may diminish complications. Unfortunately, in many larger tumours, it is clear that non-radiation factors, either intrinsic to the tumour or the host–tumour interaction, are paramount in the production of ocular complications. In this latter setting it is doubtful whether lowering radiation by using adjunctive hyperthermia will decrease complications.

A different approach to avoid radiation morbidity is to resect uveal tumours without using either brachytherapy or charged particle treatments. Even though the first use of iridocyclectomy was in 1911 and choroidectomy in 1924, there is a paucity of data (Zirm 1911, Schubert 1925, Vail 1971). Most early reports involved only single cases, and the tumours were generally quite small (Muller 1969, Vail 1971). In addition, in many reports the diagnostic error rate was quite high; even in recent reports up to 40% of tumours resected with a clinical diagnosis of uveal melanoma had another lesion on histological examination (Peyman et al 1987, Linnic 1983). Foulds, Peyman, Shields and our group have presented some cases treated with local resection (Foulds et al 1987, Shields & Shields 1988, Char 1989c). Foulds has been the pioneer in this work, and his techniques have been widely emulated (Foulds et al 1987). Surgical resection of larger uveal melanomas is technically difficult and has a substantial learning curve. Almost 30% of eyes have had to be removed after surgical resection, and this is higher than the post-radiation enucleation rate (Peyman et al 1987, Foulds et al 1987). In addition in up to 50% of eyes it is impossible to be certain that there is no tumour at the line of resection (Forrest et al 1978). Orientation and sectioning of these small specimens are difficult, and there is differential shrinkage of tumour, sclera and normal uvea. While previous investigators have shown with smaller, anterior tumours that less than 20% of such cases develop tumour recurrence, it remains to be seen what are the relative morbidities and efficacies with surgical resection versus irradiation in similar size melanomas.

A second unanswered issue is how to diminish the tumour-related mortality noted after treatment of a uveal melanoma. I suspect that most patients who develop clinically detectable metastases had microscopic systemic disease at the time of initial ocular diagnosis. Most data are consistent with the hypothesis that the initial event in the pathogenesis of most malignancies is malignant transformation of a single cell, followed by clonal expansion. It is predicted that it takes approximately 40 generations for the tumour to reach sufficient size to kill the host, and the smallest primary tumour that can be clinically detected has undergone 20 doublings (Char 1989a). It is likely that such a tumour that is in the middle or older portion of its natural history when it is first detected in the eye has already shed micrometastases.

What are appropriate trials to consider to determine if different therapies will decrease metastatic disease? One of the most important considerations in design of such a trial is to make sure that an answer can be obtained in a sufficiently short interval and that the data will be germane to state-of-the-art clinical management. A patient population must be chosen that has a high enough tumour-related mortality that a difference between two treatments can be readily detected. Uveal melanoma metastases are mainly associated with larger tumours; in our five-year follow-up after helium ion irradiation, approximately 10% of patients with tumours <16 mm in diameter and <8 mm thick developed metastatic disease (Char et al 1990). In the USA a trial is currently ongoing comparing survival after radioactive plaques and enucleation in patients with tumours of this size (Char 1989b). Given the low metastatic rate and the absence of any data that suggest better prognosis after enucleation, it is extremely doubtful whether a significant effect will be observed in that trial. Further, given these constraints it is difficult ethically to justify this trial since over 95% of patients with tumours of this size retain their eye, and many keep excellent vision. As a separate part of that study, larger tumours are being treated with either enucleation or pre-enucleation radiation and removal of the eye (Char 1989b). The latter treatment is based on studies that were initiated in 1977 (Char et al 1989c). At that time we wanted to investigate indirectly if the trauma of enucleation increased melanoma spread by seeding cells into the systemic circulation. We initiated a pre-enucleation radiation study in poor-risk patients with large uveal melanomas (20 Gy of photon irradiation one week prior to enucleation), to determine if intraocular tumour sterilization would occur and that could increase patient survival. Unfortunately, while we and others have shown that this treatment diminished both tissue culture propagation and cell cycling, it did not improve survival (Char et al 1989c, Kreissig et al 1989, Bornfeld et al 1989). In our experience, survival was significantly worse in the pre-enucleation radiation group (Char et al 1989c). Our study was retrospective; however, the control patients were operated on by the same surgeon, and were chosen from patients with similar size tumours that were managed in our oncology unit in the 24 months prior to the inception of either charged particle or pre-enucleation radiation trials. The choice of that control group diminished the possibility of treatment selection bias.

Since many patients who develop widespread disease have clinically undetectable metastases at the time of ocular diagnosis, adjunctive therapy at the time of ocular therapy is reasonable; however, a number of problems exist. In one small retrospective study it appeared that the adjunctive multi-drug chemotherapy may have decreased tumour-related mortality; however, only 20 patients were analysed (Sellami et al 1986). There are significant complications associated with any form of chemotherapy, and metastatic melanoma response rates with current agents are too low to consider such a trial (Voigt & Kleeberg 1984). A number of newer agents are being evaluated in phase I–II studies, and it is likely that one of these will be used to treat poor-risk uveal melanoma patients at the time of enucleation.

There are a number of different approaches being used to treat metastatic melanoma. Traditional single or multi-drug chemotherapy has generally shown approximately a 25% partial response rate in metastatic skin or uveal melanoma. Chemo-embolization of the liver for hepatic metastases has been effective in up to 50% of uveal melanoma patients (Mavligit et al 1988). In cutaneous metastatic melanoma, excellent responses have been observed with interleukin-2 lymphocyte-activated killer (LAK) cells (Rosenberg et al 1988). Unfortunately the response in metastatic uveal melanoma has not been good with this protocol (unpublished data). A number of investigators have used murine monoclonal antibodies directed towards tumour-associated antigens to diagnose both primary and metastatic retinoblastoma and uveal melanoma (Herlyn et al 1987, Schroff et al 1987, Furukawa et al 1989). Unfortunately there are a number of problems associated with the use of monoclonal antibodies. There are very few tumour-associated antigens that are unique to a tumour, and antigens shared between normal and tumour cells are common. Often antigen expression on a primary neoplasm is different from the expression of the same patient's metastatic foci. The vascular supply to a tumour may be poor and it is difficult to develop strategies to deliver antibody or antibody-toxic substrates to such metastases. Finally, the use of murine monoclonal antibodies therapeutically is problematic since the host begins to eliminate these agents within 30 minutes and becomes sensitized to the murine antigens on the second injection. For these and other reasons the efficacies with immunotherapy in the treatment of human metastases has been relatively limited.

A number of newer approaches are being used, but at present we have not had sufficient experience in uveal metastatic melanoma to determine their potential.

It is likely in the future that we will treat high-risk uveal melanoma patients with systemic adjunctive therapy at the time their ocular tumour is diagnosed and managed. Unfortunately at present we are unable to do this, and for that reason most patients probably have micrometastases at the time of initial ocular presentation and are not cured by ocular intervention alone.

ACKNOWLEDGEMENTS

This work was supported in part by NIH grant EYO 7504, American Cancer Society grant PDT-321, NIH-NCI CA 19138, DOE DE-AC03-76SF00098, and by unrestricted grants from That Man May See, the Weltkunst Foundation, and Research to Prevent Blindness.

REFERENCES

Abe M, Hiraoka M 1985 Localized hyperthermia and radiation in cancer therapy. Int J Radiat Biol 47: 347

Augsburger J J, Gamel J W, Shields J A et al 1987 Post-irradiation regression of choroidal melanomas as a risk factor for death from metastatic disease. Ophthalmology 94: 1173–1177

Bedford M A, Bedotto C, MacFaul P A 1970 Radiation retinopathy after the application of a cobalt plaque. Br J Ophthalmol 54: 505–509

Blakely E A, Lyman J T, Chen G T Y et al 1985 Radiobiological studies for helium ion therapy of uveal melanoma. Int J Radiat Oncology Biol Phys 11 (suppl 1): 134

Boone M L M, Lawrence J H, Connor W G et al 1977 Introductions to the use of protons and heavy ions in radiation therapy: historical perspective. Int J Radiat Oncol Biol Phys 3: 65–69

Bornfeld N, Huser U, Sauerwein W et al 1989 Praoperative Bestrahlung vor Enukleation bei malignem Melanom der Uvea. Klin Monatsbl Augenheilkd 194: 252

Bosworth J L, Packer S, Rotman M et al 1988 Choroidal melanoma: I-125 plaque therapy. Radiology 169: 249

Brady L W, Markoe A M, Amendola B E et al 1988 The treatment of primary intraocular malignancy. Int J Radiat Oncol Biol Phys 15: 1355–1361

Brovkina A F, Zarubei G D 1986 Ciliochoroidal melanomas treated with a narrow medical proton beam. Arch Ophthalmol 104: 402–404

Bujara K, Hallerman D 1984 Netzhaut-Aderhautnarbe nach Bestrahlung eines malignen Melanoms der Aderhaut mit dem Ruthenium-106-Applikator. Ophthalmologica 188: 29–34

Busse H, Muller R-P, Kroll P 1983 Results of ^{106}Ru/^{106}Rh radiation of choroidal melanomas. Am J Ophthalmol 15: 1146–1149

Cappin J M 1973 Malignant melanoma and rubeosis iridis: histopathological and statistical study. Br J Ophthalmol 57: 815

Char D H 1984 Therapeutic options in uveal melanoma. Am J Ophthalmol 98: 796–799

Char D H 1989a Clinical ocular oncology. Churchill Livingstone, Edinburgh

Char D H 1989b Current treatments and trials in uveal melanoma. Oncology 3: 113–121

Char D H 1989c Eyewall resection and radiation for anterior melanomas. Trans Soc Acad Ophthalmol (submitted for publication)

Char D H, Lonn L, Margolis L 1977 Complications of cobalt plaque therapy of choroidal melanomas. Am J Ophthalmol 84. 536–541

Char D H, Castro J R, Quivey J M et al 1980 Helium ion charged particle therapy for choroidal melanoma. Ophthalmology 87: 565–570

Char D H, Huhta K, Waldman F 1989a DNA cell cycle studies in uveal melanoma. Am J Ophthalmol 107: 65–72

Char D H, Castro J R, Quivey J M et al 1989b Uveal melanoma radiation: ^{125}I versus helium ion irradiation. Ophthalmology 96: 1708–1715

Char D H, Crawford J B, Kaleta-Michaels S et al 1989c Analysis of radiation failure after uveal melanoma brachytherapy. Am J Ophthalmol 108: 712–716

Char D H, Castro J R, Kroll S M et al 1990 Five-year follow-up of helium ion therapy. Ophthalmology 108: 209–214

Chuvilo I V, Goldin L L, Khoroshkov V S et al 1984 ITEP synchronotron proton beam in radiotherapy. Int J Radiat Oncol Biol Phys 10: 185–195

Coleman D J, Lizzi F L, Burgess S E P et al 1986 Ultrasonic hyperthermia and radiation in the management of intraocular malignant melanoma. Am J Ophthalmol 101: 635

Constable I J, Koehler A M, Schmidt R E 1975 Proton irradiation of simulated ocular tumors. Invest Ophthalmol Vis Sci 14: 547–555

Crawford J B, Char D H 1987 Histopathology of uveal melanomas treated with charged particle radiation. Ophthalmology 94: 639–643

Egan K M, Gragoudas E S, Seddon J M 1989 The risk of enucleation after proton beam irradiation of uveal melanoma. Ophthalmology 96: 1377–1383

Finger P T, Packer S, Paglione R W et al 1989 Thermoradiotherapy of choroidal melanoma. Ophthalmology 96: 1384

Forrest A W, Keyser R B, Spencer W H 1978 Iridocyclectomy for melanomas of the ciliary body: a follow up study of pathology and surgical morbidity. Trans Am Acad Ophthalmol Otolaryngol 85: 1237

Foulds W S, Damato B E, Burton R L 1987 Local resection versus enucleation in the management of choroidal melanoma. Eye 1: 676

Furukawa K S, Furukawa K, Real F X 1989 A unique antigenic epitope of human melanomas carried on the common melanoma glycoprotein gp^{95}/p^{97}. J Exp Med 169: 585

Gass J D 1985 Comparison of prognosis after enucleation vs cobalt 60 irradiation of melanomas. Arch Ophthalmol 103: 916

Glynn R J, Seddon J M, Gragoudas E S et al 1989 Evaluation of tumour regression and other prognostic factors for early and late metastasis after proton irradiation of uveal melanoma. Ophthalmology 96: 1566–1573

Goitein M, Miller T 1983 Planning proton therapy of the eye. Med Phys 10: 275–283

Goodman D, Char D H, Crawford J B et al 1986 Uveal melanoma necrosis following helium ion therapy. Am J Ophthalmol 101: 643–645

Gragoudas E S, Goitein M, Koehler A M et al 1977 Proton irradiation of small choroidal malignant melanomas. Am J Ophthalmol 83: 665–673

Gragoudas E S, Seddon J M, Egan K et al 1987 Long-term results of proton beam irradiated uveal melanomas. Ophthalmology 94: 349–353

Gragoudas E S, Seddon J M, Egan K M et al 1988 Metastasis from uveal melanoma after proton beam irradiation. Ophthalmology 95: 992–999

Herlyn M, Rodeck U, Mancianti M L et al 1987 Expression of melanoma-associated antigens in rapidly dividing human melanocytes in culture. Cancer Res 47: 3057

Kim M K, Char D H, Castro J R et al 1986 Neovascular glaucoma after helium ion irradiation for uveal melanoma. Ophthalmology 93: 189–193

Kindy-Degnan N, Char D H, Castro J R et al 1989 Effect of various doses of radiation for uveal melanoma on regression, visual acuity, complications, and survival. Am J Ophthalmol 107: 114–120

Kreissig I, Rohrbach M, Lincoff H 1989 Irradiation of choroidal melanomas before enucleation? Retina 9: 101

Lawton A W 1989 Proton beam therapy for uveal melanoma. Opthalmology 96: 138

Linnic L F 1983 Surgical treatment of melanomas of the iris, ciliary body and choroid. In: Lommatzsch P K, Blodi F C (eds) Intraocular tumours. Akademie Verlag, Berlin, pp 409–416

Linstadt D, Char D H, Castro J R et al 1988 Vision following helium ion radiotherapy of uveal melanoma: a Northern California Group Study. Int J Radiat Oncol Biol Phys 15: 347–352

Lommatzsch P K 1983 Beta-irradiation of choroidal melanoma with $^{106}Ru/^{106}Rh$ applicators. Arch Ophthalmol 101: 713–717

MacFaul P A 1977 Local radiotherapy in the treatment of malignant melanoma of the choroid. Trans Ophthalmol Soc UK 97: 421–427

MacFaul P A, Bedford M A 1970 Ocular complications after therapeutic irradiation. Br J

Ophthalmol 54: 237–247

Manschot W A, Van Strik R 1987 Is irradiation a justifiable treatment of choroidal melanoma? Analysis of published results. Br J Ophthalmol 71: 348–352

Mavligit G M, Charnsangavej C, Carrasco H 1988 Regression of ocular melanoma metastatic to the liver after hepatic arterial chemoembolization with cisplatin and polyvinyl sponge. JAMA 260: 974

Moore R F 1930 Choroidal sarcoma treated by the intra-ocular insertion of radon seeds. Br J Ophthalmol 14: 145–152

Muller H K 1969 Die Partielle Ausschneidung von Iris und Ciliarkorper. Doc Ophthalol 26: 279

Oosterhuis J A, Lommatsch P K, Wessing A 1988 Is radiation justifiable treatment of choroidal melanoma? Br J Ophthalmol 72: 317–318

Paliwal B R, Shrivastava P N, Haney P 1989 Hyperthermia: principles and quality assurance. Med Dosim 14: 117–123

Perez C A, Gillespie B, Pajak T et al 1989 Quality assurance problems in clinical hyperthermia and their impact on therapeutic outcome: a report by the radiation therapy oncology group. Int J Radiat Oncol Biol Phys 16: 551

Peyman G A, Schulman J, Raichand M 1987 Diagnosis and therapeutic surgery of the uvea. Part two: results. Ophthalmic Surg 18: 310

Rosenberg S A, Lotze M T, Mule J J 1988 New approaches to the immunotherapy of cancer using interleukin-2. Ann Int Med 108: 853

Schroff R W, Morgan A C Jr, Woodhouse C S et al 1987 Monoclonal antibody therapy in malignant melanoma: factors effecting in vivo localization. J Biol Modif 6: 457–472

Schubert F 1925 Operation eines 'Leucosarkoms' der choroididea mit Erhaltung des Auges: Dauerheilung. Wien Klin Wochenschr 30: 677–678

Seddon J M, Gragoudas E S, Albert D M et al 1985 Comparison of survival rates for patients with uveal melanoma after treatment with proton beam irradiation or enucleation. Am J Ophthalmol 99: 282–290

Sellami M, Weil M, Dhermy P et al 1986 Adjuvant chemotherapy in ocular melanoma: study of 20 cases. Oncology 43: 221–223

Shields J A, Shields C L 1988 Surgical approach to lamellar sclerouvectomy for posterior uveal melanoma: the 1986 Schoenberg Lecture. Ophthalmic Surg 19: 774

Stallard H B 1933 Radiant energy as (a) a pathogenic (b) a therapeutic agent in ocular disorders. Br J Ophthalmol (suppl) 7: 70

Stallard H B 1959 Malignant melanoma of the choroid treated with radioactive applicators. Trans Ophthalmol Soc UK 79: 373–392

Stallard H B 1961 Malignant melanoma of the choroid treated with radioactive applicators. J R Coll Surg Edinb 29: 170–182

Stallard II B 1968 Malignant melanoblastoma of the choroid. Mod Probl Ophthalmol 7: 16–38

Suit II D, Gallagher H S 1964 Intact tumour cells in irradiated tissue. Arch Pathol 78: 648–651

Tobias C A 1985 The future of heavy-ion science in biology of medicine. Radiat Res 103: 133

Tolmach L J 1961 Growth patterns in x-irradiated HeLa cells. Ann NY Acad Sci 95: 743–757

Vail D T 1971 Iridocyclectomy: a review. Am J Ophthalmol 71: 161

Voigt H, Kleeberg U R 1984 Pala, Vindesine, and cisplatin combination chemotherapy in advanced malignant melanoma. Cancer 53: 2058–2062

Zirm E 1911 Ubert endobulbare Operationen. Arch Augenheilkd 69: 233

Zografos L, Gailloud C, Perret C et al 1988 Report on the conservative treatment of melanoma of the uvea at the Lausanne University Ophthalmologic Clinic. Klin Monatsbl Augenheilkd 192: 572–578

11

Molecular genetics in clinical ophthalmology

B. Jay   M. Jay

INTRODUCTION

Recent advances in molecular genetics are producing fundamental changes in our understanding and practice of medicine which are both exciting and important. In order to help ophthalmologists understand these advances, we are describing here some of the techniques that are applied in molecular biology, and are illustrating the use of these techniques in X-linked ophthalmic disorders, Leber's hereditary optic neuropathy and retinoblastoma.

TECHNIQUES IN MOLECULAR BIOLOGY

Basic concepts

DNA has been called the molecule of life, and it constitutes the template which governs cellular replication. DNA molecules consist of two strands of nucleotide bases joined by hydrogen bonds to form a double helix. Each strand is formed by a sequence of any one of four bases, adenine (A), guanine (G), cytosine (C) and thymine (T), joined to a sugar (deoxyribose) and a phosphate. The bonding between bases links the two strands in such a way that A always pairs with T, and G always pairs with C and reciprocally. If the sequence of bases along one strand is known, then the sequence along the complementary strand can be inferred. The sequence of bases along one strand forms the genetic code, since each triplet determines an amino acid. DNA is transcribed into a ribonucleic acid called messenger RNA (mRNA), and it is mRNA which moves from the nucleus to the cytoplasm, where it acts as the blueprint for protein synthesis.

The structure of mRNA is very similar to that of DNA but it differs in two respects. mRNA is single stranded; it is complementary to one strand of DNA but the base uracil (U) is substituted for thymine (T). It differs also from DNA in that there are intervening sequences of DNA known as introns which are spliced out when RNA is transcribed, and the remaining sequences known as exons form the basis of mRNA (Fig. 11.1).

Much of DNA consists of highly repetitive sequences which, like introns, are thought not to have any function, so that only a certain proportion of DNA can be considered to consist of genes. It is estimated that the human

185

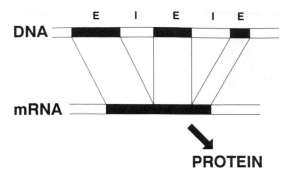

Fig. 11.1   Showing loss of introns (I) when DNA is transcribed into mRNA, the mRNA consisting largely of exons (E).

genome, the total amount of DNA in the nucleus of each cell, consists of about 3×10^9 base pairs and that there may be about 10 000 genes.

Much of the manipulation of DNA in the laboratory depends on two of its properties. The first is that DNA can be cleaved in a reproducible manner by the use of certain enzymes known as restriction enzymes (Roberts 1985). These enzymes are endonucleases, for the most part derived from bacterial organisms, which recognize a specific sequence of DNA, usually of the order of four to ten base pairs and which cleave DNA at some point in that sequence. Each restriction enzyme has its own specific recognition sequence or cleavage site and will always cleave DNA in the same way, generating fragments of various lengths (Fig. 11.2). The second property of DNA which is used in the laboratory is its ability to form hybrids in certain conditions. DNA from one individual can be separated into its constituent strands by a process of denaturing, either by heating to 95°C or by treatment with alkali. If single-stranded DNA from another source is then introduced, the two

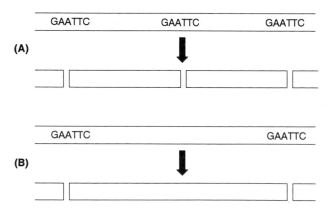

Fig. 11.2   The restriction enzyme EcoRI recognizes the sequence of bases GAATTC, and cleaves this sequence between G and A. The loss of a cleavage site in **B** results in larger fragments of DNA than in **A**.

DNAs from different origins will form a hybrid, provided their sequences of base pairs are complementary. These two properties form the basis of a technique used to analyse genes, a technique called Southern blotting (Southern 1975).

Southern blotting

DNA is isolated from a blood sample and cleaved with a restriction enzyme. This generates hundreds of thousands of fragments of DNA which are then separated according to size by gel electrophoresis. The smaller fragments travel faster through the gel, the larger fragments remaining nearer the top. The whole gel is then blotted on to a nitrocellulose filter and the strands are denatured. The filter thereby retains the pattern of single-stranded fragments of DNA according to their size. At this point cloned DNA, which has been radioactively labelled and which is known as a probe, is now applied. A probe is so named because it is a short sequence of single-stranded DNA which will select any sequence complementary to it among the fragments on the filter, and will hybridize with such sequences. The excess of probe which has not hybridized is washed off, and autoradiography on X-ray film will reveal any hybrids as bands (or Southern blots). It is the analysis of the patterns of these blots which forms the basis of much of gene mapping, and many of the methods used depend on the choice of probes.

Probes

There are three main types of probe. These are gene-specific probes, oligonucleotide probes and probes recognizing variation. Gene-specific probes are used where the gene product is known, as for example factor VIII in classical haemophilia (Gitschier et al 1985). It is possible to work from the protein sequence in the gene product, to the amino acid sequence, and to construct the corresponding mRNA. Under the action of an enzyme known as reverse transcriptase, the mRNA is copied to single-stranded DNA, which in turn, and with the use of the enzyme DNA polymerase, acts as a primer for the synthesis of a complementary strand; the result is a molecule known as cDNA (DNA complementary to the mRNA). This cDNA can be cloned, labelled radioactively and used in Southern blotting. The pattern of the blots obtained is shown to be different in normal and affected individuals, and is due to the presence, or the absence, of an abnormality of the gene product.

Another group of probes are the oligonucleotide probes and, as the name implies, these are short sequences of DNA usually of the order of 15–30 bases and which correspond to a sequence which is known to occur in the gene. Oligonucleotide probes recognize point mutations which involve the substitution of one base for another within these particular sequences (Wallace et al 1981).

The third group of probes are those which recognize variation in the form of DNA polymorphisms. In addition to much of DNA containing non-coding sequences, much of DNA is also polymorphic, that is to say that alternative forms exist. It is estimated that about one base in 150 is polymorphic, that is, it can exist as any one of the four bases A, T, G or C. As a consequence, some of these polymorphic sites occur within a cleavage site of a restriction enzyme and result in the loss of a cleavage site. It follows that these polymorphisms affect the size of fragments generated by cleavage, and they are therefore termed restriction fragment length polymorphisms or RFLPs. Due to an RFLP, two given fragments from a pair of homologous chromosomes will be either of the same length, or of different lengths (Fig. 11.3). Individuals are therefore homozygous or heterozygous for an RFLP which can be considered as a two-allele system and which is transmitted in a Mendelian fashion. Probes which detect an RFLP are usually sequences of DNA taken from a known source or chromosome and which are near a polymorphic site. There are other probes detecting variation known as variable number of tandem repeats (VNTR) (Jeffreys et al 1985). These tandem repeats are very short sequences of DNA, usually between two and 80 base pairs in length, which are repeated either in a head-to-tail or in a back-to-back fashion. The distance between two cleavage sites containing VNTRs varies according to the number of repeats, and probes may be selected which detect this variation. VNTR probes are also known as mini-satellite probes, and they have the advantage that they are highly polymorphic, so that there is great variation among individuals, and the proportion of people in the population who are heterozygous for this multi-allele system is far higher than those heterozygous for RFLPs.

Preparation of probes

The construction of gene-specific probes has already been described, but other probes are constructed on the principle that they must be sequences of DNA from a known source, and each sequence must be present in a large quantity. Sequences of DNA from a known source may be selected either from somatic cell hybrids (reviewed by Ruddle 1981), or by chromosome isolation using a fluorescence-activated cell sorter (FACS).

Somatic cell hybrids have been used in gene mapping since 1967, when it was found that under certain laboratory conditions it is possible to fuse nuclei of cells of two species, usually human and rodent cells. In subsequent cell

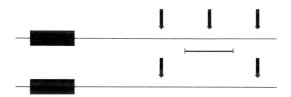

Fig. 11.3 Showing two homologous chromosomes with the locus of the gene of interest upstream (black box). The arrows indicate cleavage sites and illustrate an RFLP. This RFLP is detected by a probe which is shown as a short line in the region of the polymorphism.

culture, these hybrid cells lose human chromosomes, and finally retain only one human chromosome. The presence of a human protein in the hybrid cell is then correlated with the presence of a particular human chromosome. Hybrid cell lines containing a given chromosome can therefore be used as a source of material for probes.

Another method of isolating chromosomes is the use of a fluorescence-activated cell sorter (FACS), a machine which uses a laser to sort chromosomes according to their fluorescence (Davies et al 1981). Chromosomes are stained with ethidium bromide which makes them fluoresce, and each chromosome has its own fluorescence profile which depends on its DNA content.

The next step in the process of producing probes is to amplify the amount of DNA obtained from a given chromosome. This is done by molecular cloning using a vector, which is a vehicle for cloning. DNA from a chosen chromosome is cleaved with a restriction enzyme and inserted into vectors – usually plasmids, cosmids or phage. Plasmids are circular DNA which will accept an insert of foreign DNA and which can be cloned in bacteria. Cosmids and phage are similar to plasmids and are selected according to the size of the insert of foreign DNA which is required. A collection of clones with at least one copy of every DNA sequence in a chromosome is known as a chromosome library, and similarly there are genomic libraries. Probes are selected at random from clones, and are tested against a panel of DNAs from a number of normals. Those probes which detect variation are those which are finally chosen, and these probes are used in linkage (see Ott 1986 for a review of the principles of linkage).

Linkage

Two genes are linked if their locus, or chromosome location, is on the same chromosome. The first step in gene mapping is to find a chromosome location, or marker, which is physically close to the disease locus so that the presence of the marker implies the presence of the disease locus. RFLPs constitute a marker system which is of value providing the polymorphism is sufficiently close to the gene of interest. At meiosis, homologous chromosomes exchange segments in a process called recombination (Fig. 11.4). The order of genes is altered and genes which are close together will tend to remain undisturbed on the same chromosome, but genes which are further apart may become separated from each other and end on separate chromosomes. The frequency of recombination between two genes, or between one gene and a marker, is a measure of the distance between them. By convention, 1% of recombination is equal to a unit called the centimorgan (cM), and the centimorgan is equivalent approximately to the megabase (Mb) (1 Mb is equal to 1000 kilobases (kb) or 1 000 000 base pairs (bp)). The other parameter used in linkage is the lod score, which is a logarithm of the odds (or probability)

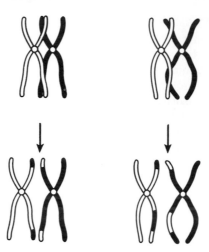

Fig. 11.4   Crossing over or recombination. The maternally and paternally derived chromosomes exchange segments at meiosis.

of linkage. A lod score is calculated for each pedigree and for a given recombination fraction. Linkage is significant if the lod score, represented by the letter z, is equal to or greater than 3. This corresponds to odds of 1000 : 1 in favour of linkage. Linkage is excluded for values of z less than 2. The advantage of using logarithms is that these are additive when calculating probabilities of linkage using data pooled from several pedigrees. It is often the case in gene mapping that data are pooled from several studies, since the disorder studied may be rare and there is only a finite number of suitable families for DNA linkage. In practice, linkage is first found to one marker or RFLP identifying a chromosomal locus. The notation which is used for probes is somewhat haphazard and based on laboratory bench numbers or even the initials of researchers. A probe, however, identifies an RFLP whose locus is designated by a precise combination of letters and numbers: 'D' for DNA, followed by the chromosome number or the letter X or Y for a sex chromosome, 'S' or 'Z' for single or repeat sequence, and finally a number which corresponds to the chronological order in which the loci on the relevant chromosome have been mapped. Linkage to one marker is found first, and followed by linkage to several markers in the same region. The order of these markers relative to the disease locus is calculated by a process called multi-point linkage and which requires the use of a computer program. The result is a map which gives the genetic distance between markers and the disease locus. The actual physical distance between markers may not be the same as the genetic distance, and this is due to the fact that the frequency of recombination is not constant along a chromosome. Physical distances are determined using other methods, one of which is pulsed field gel electrophoresis.

Pulsed field gel electrophoresis (PFGE)

Conventional electrophoresis is a process in which an electrical field is used to move DNA fragments through an agarose gel. The rate at which the fragments move depends on their size, and this method is used for fragments which do not exceed 20–30 kb. A development of this method is PFGE, which can separate fragments which are between 50 kb and 10 000 kb in size (reviewed by Barlow 1989). DNA is cleaved with restriction fragments which are chosen for having rare cutting sites, and this generates fragments of large size. These fragments are separated by gel electrophoresis in which the electrical pulse is applied in two perpendicular directions, and in which the duration of the pulse is varied. The gel can now be used for Southern blotting in the same way as in conventional electrophoresis.

This technique is one way of constructing a long-range restriction map of a region of interest. If DNA from a specific region is subjected to successive cleavage by different restriction enzymes, and fragments separated by gel electrophoresis, the relative order of the cleavage sites can be inferred. These sites are arranged in order and represent a map which covers a chromosome region. PFGE is used to construct such a map by identifying any two probes which hybridize to the same fragment, since the probes will therefore be separated by a distance which is no greater than the length of the fragment. A map of probes and the physical distance between them can be constructed. The aim is to find markers flanking the gene which are separated by no more than 1 Mb and identified by a particular fragment on a PFGE gel. It is then possible to cut that fragment out of the gel and use the DNA to create a library of clones of the region of interest. It is also possible to amplify a PFGE fragment by molecular cloning using an appropriate vector, in this case yeast artificial chromosomes which are capable of accepting large inserts. Amplification of much shorter sequences of DNA, of the order of 1 kb, is achieved by the use of the polymerase chain reaction technique.

Polymerase chain reaction (PCR)

The PCR requires two flanking sequences to the sequence which is being amplified (Saiki et al 1988). Short sequences of about 20 bp are constructed from these flanking sequences and act as primers which are mixed with the target DNA. A heat-stable enzyme, Taq polymerase, is used, and the ingredients mixed with the four nucleotides (A, C, T, G). Heating separates the target DNA into its two strands, the primers then anneal to each end and the target sequence is synthesized. This constitutes one cycle during which the amount of target DNA is doubled (Fig. 11.5). Repeated cycles double the quantity at each cycle, and the reaction is usually run 30 times, which amplifies the target DNA by 10^5 to 10^6 fold. Much of this process is now automated and allows rapid results in many different types of DNA analysis including prenatal diagnosis.

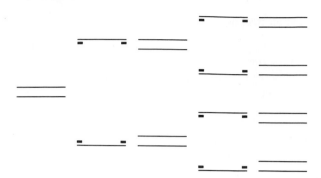

Fig. 11.5 Showing the polymerase chain reaction. The short sequence of DNA (shown on the far left) is denatured, primers (small black boxes) are annealed and initiate the synthesis of the complementary sequence of DNA. The figure shows how four copies of one sequence are obtained in the first two steps of a PCR.

Chromosome walking and jumping

In gene mapping, a situation will arise when a more precise characterization of a DNA sequence of about 80 kb or more is needed. The principle is to construct a library of clones by cleaving the entire genome and cloning the fragments, and then to identify a clone taken from the library which contains a known marker such as an RFLP. That clone will act as the start of a walk into the unknown contiguous fragments. The clone at the start of the walk is cleaved into smaller fragments which are then subcloned. One of the subcloned fragments is then used as a probe to screen the library, and this will select the adjacent clone. Using this technique, the DNA sequence of interest can be characterized in terms of overlapping clones of a size of the order of 15 kb. There are drawbacks to this strategy and these are due to the fact that (a) the 'walk' has to be in both directions, and (b) the 'walk' may come to a halt if highly repetitive sequence of DNA is reached. This latter drawback may be overcome by using chromosome jumping, which is an extension of the same principle as chromosome walking. In chromosome jumping, libraries are generated using restriction enzymes which cleave at rare cutting sites, thus generating larger fragments, one of which may hopefully contain the gene of interest. These larger fragments are cloned and are used in chromosome jumping in the same way as smaller clones are used in chromosome walking.

The potentials for the application of molecular biology to all branches of clinical medicine are enormous, and hopefully will lead to exciting advances in many aspects of ophthalmology. For those interested in reading further on this subject, the works of Weatherall (1985), Davies (1988) and Kingston (1989) can be recommended.

THE X CHROMOSOME AND THE EYE

Many of the earliest applications of molecular genetics were in the study of X-linked disorders, partly because the very characteristic mode of inheritance identified the X chromosome as being the site of the gene locus, thus obviating a search throughout the 22 autosomes, and partly because the X chromosome contained a large number of polymorphic sites which could be used for linkage studies. We will look at a number of X-linked conditions of interest to ophthalmologists and the advances that have occurred in understanding their genetic basis.

X-linked retinitis pigmentosa (XLRP)

XLRP is one of the more severe forms of this heterogeneous group of disorders, occurring in 15–20% of index patients in Britain (Jay 1982, Bundey & Crews 1984). In affected (hemizygous) males it produces symptoms of night blindness from childhood, considerable constriction of the visual fields by early adult life, and blindness usually by the age of 40 years. Occasional families appear to have a milder form of the disease; it is not yet known whether these patients have a mutation allelic with one of the two already identified (see below) or a mutation at a third locus.

In 1984 the gene responsible for XLRP was mapped to the short arm of the X chromosome. The initial report (Bhattacharya et al 1984) was of close linkage of XLRP to the polymorphism DXS7, identified with the probe L1.28, which maps to band 11.3 on the short arm of the X chromosome (Xp11.3). Several subsequent reports suggested, however, that there may be a more distal site for XLRP at Xp21 (Nussbaum et al 1985a, Francke et al 1985, Denton et al 1988), and that families with a scintillating golden-metallic sheen (tapetal reflex) in the fundi of carriers had a form of XLRP that mapped distal to DXS7.

Support for this more distal site resulted from studying two boys with deletion syndromes. In one boy with Duchenne muscular dystrophy, chronic granulomatous disease (CGD), McLeod phenotype and retinitis pigmentosa, an interstitial deletion of part of Xp21 was identified (Francke et al 1985), a deletion at an appreciable distance from Xp11.3, the site of the originally described locus for XLRP. In the second boy CGD, McLeod phenotype and retinitis pigmentosa (Saint-Basile et al 1988) could be explained by the occurrence of a microdeletion involving these loci. His mother displayed mild abnormalities in her fundi, consistent with the diagnosis of the carrier state of X-linked retinitis pigmentosa. In the affected boy, markers close to Xp11.3 (754, L1.28, 2bA3 and OTC) were all present, but the CGD gene in the Xp21 region was deleted. Unless the gene deletion in this patient is part of a more complex rearrangement, the occurrence of CGD, McLeod phenotype and XLRP would support localization of these genes to Xp21, as in the patient reported by Francke et al (1985). These findings argue for there being two loci for XLRP, and this heterogeneity was accepted at the 9th Human Gene Mapping Workshop (HGM9 1987) when the proximal locus in band Xp11.3–p11.2 was designated RP2 and the distal locus in band Xp21.1 p21.4 was designated RP3 (Fig. 11.6).

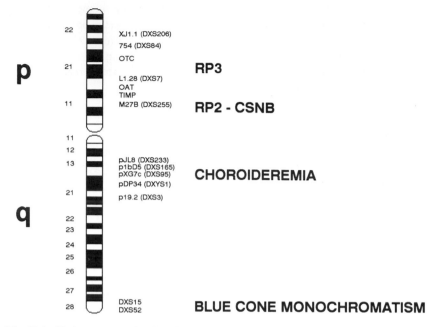

Fig. 11.6 X chromosome showing sites of the two retinitis pigmentosa genes, RP2 and RP3 on the short arm 'p'. The sites of the genes for congenital stationary night blindness (CSNB), choroideremia and blue cone monochromatism, the last two loci being on the long arm 'q', are also shown, as are the sites of most of the probes and loci mentioned in the text.

The family previously reported by Nussbaum et al (1985a) was studied further when the carrier females were found to have a metallic sheen in their fundi. The XLRP locus showed close linkage with Xp21 marker loci OTC and DXS206 (Musarella et al 1989a). In one family from Northern Ireland, the RP gene appeared to be located between XJ1.1 and M27β (Redmond et al 1990), but unlike other reports of families with RP3 (Friedrich et al 1985, Denton et al 1988) none of the females in this Irish family exhibited a tapetal reflex.

The evidence at present available suggests that in families where a tapetal reflex is seen in carrier females this indicates the RP3 gene; its absence is unhelpful in distinguishing between the RP2 and RP3 genes.

At the present time about one half of families are informative for a probe linked to one or other locus, and this information has been used for genetic counselling and prenatal diagnosis.

Congenital stationary night blindness (CSNB)

The complete form of CSNB is characterized by non-progressive night blindness from birth, subnormal visual acuity, myopia and normal fundi.

Children may present with nystagmus and subnormal vision and the importance of making the correct diagnosis is that this is a stationary condition, not a progressive retinal dystrophy. These patients have a Schubert–Bornschein or negative-type electroretinogram (ERG), with no demonstrable scotopic rod-mediated ERG b-wave, and the oscillatory potentials are markedly reduced (Miyake et al 1986).

Seven out of eight families with CSNB demonstrate close linkage with DXS7 and looser linkage with tissue inhibitor of metalloproteinase (TIMP) and DXS255, all of which are in Xp11 (Musarella et al 1989b), as is the RP2 gene. In three other families with CSNB similar close linkage to DXS7 was observed (Gal et al 1989) and it remains to be seen whether the genes for the complete form of CSNB and RP2 are allelic.

Norrie disease

Affected males with Norrie disease are blind from birth; one-third have an appreciable hearing loss and one-quarter are psychotic and appear mentally retarded. Histological examination of the eye shows retinal dysplasia, abundant vascular proliferation and haemorrhages. Carrier females have normal fundi.

Close linkage has been demonstrated between Norrie disease and the locus DXS7 as defined by the TaqI RFLP detected with the probe L1.28 (Gal et al 1985a, 1985b, Bleeker-Wagemakers et al 1985, Kivlin et al 1987). Recombination between the gene for Norrie disease and L1.28 has been described (Katayama et al 1988, Ngo et al 1988a), and it has been suggested that there may be about a 4% error rate introduced by meiotic crossovers in carriers on prenatal diagnosis based on linkage between Norrie disease and DXS7 (Katayama et al 1988).

Both the Norrie disease and DXS7 loci are included in small submicroscopic interstitial deletions of the X chromosome in three independent families (Gal et al 1985a, 1986, de la Chapelle et al 1985, Forrest et al 1987), and the exclusion of Norrie disease was confirmed by demonstrating the DXS7 DNA sequence in a fetus (de la Chapelle et al 1985). The DXS7 locus, together with the monoamine oxidase A and B genes, was deleted in another patient with Norrie disease, adding further confirmation that these loci are close together, the deletion involving band Xp11.3 (Lan et al 1989).

Using human ornithine aminotransferase (OAT) cDNA which recognizes OAT-related sequences in the same region of the X chromosome as the L1.28 probe (Barrett et al 1987), an RFLP of 4.8 kb in size was found. In the family reported by Ngo et al (1988a), this fragment was not expressed in affected males but was in obligate heterozygotes and normal males. This finding suggests linkage between this locus and the Norrie disease locus (Ngo et al 1988b, 1989), thus making the OAT-like gene sequences a good candidate for a DNA marker for the disease.

Choroideremia

Choroideremia, like X-linked retinitis pigmentosa, presents in childhood with night blindness, but thereafter the course of choroideremia is slower, with field defects becoming apparent in young adults, and useful central vision usually being preserved into the sixth decade of life. Carrier females tend to have a characteristic fundus appearance, with deep retinal pigmentation often in a linear distribution in the mid-periphery, associated with spotty pigment epithelial atrophy. Choroideremia may be difficult to distinguish from XLRP, but the presence of a carrier female with characteristic fundus changes makes the distinction easier.

The gene locus for choroideremia has been assigned to the proximal long arm of the X chromosome through demonstration of tight linkage with various RFLPs located in the Xq13–q21 region (Nussbaum et al 1985b, Schwartz et al 1986, Sankila et al 1987, Lesko et al 1987). Recombinations between choroideremia and DXYS1 and DXS3, two of the loci in this part of the long arm of the X chromosome, have been reported and this suggests that linkage is not as close as had previously been suggested (MacDonald et al 1987).

Deletions spanning part of Xq21 are associated with choroideremia and mental retardation, deafness being another common feature (Nussbaum et al 1987, Schwartz et al 1986, Hodgson et al 1987, Cremers et al 1990). In two patients a deletion of the DXS165 locus and (part of) the choroideremia gene were demonstrated (Cremers et al 1987), while more extensive studies have assigned the choroideremia locus to Xq21, spanning the loci DXS95, DXS165 and DXS233 (Cremers et al 1989). In two patients with choroideremia and X-linked deafness with stapes fixation and perilymphatic gushing (DFN3), the overlapping deletions included DXS233 and DXS95 (Merry et al 1989).

These recent studies have resulted in the majority of families with choroideremia being informative, and confirmation of the carrier state, more accurate genetic counselling and prenatal diagnosis are now all possible in this condition.

Colour vision and its defects

Advances in molecular genetics have increased our understanding of the genes encoding visual pigments. This in turn has given us new insight into the mechanisms of normal and abnormal colour vision.

Visual pigments consist of an apoprotein, opsin, linked to 11-*cis*-retinal, the apoprotein in each of the visual pigments being encoded by a different gene. The absorption of a photon by a visual pigment results in the isomerization of retinal from the 11-*cis* to the all-*trans* configuration and this ultimately results in the production of a neural signal.

Recent work by Nathans et al (1986a, 1986b) started with the assumption that the rod pigment rhodopsin and the cone pigments all evolved from a common ancestor and, as a result, would contain similar sequences of nucleotides. Using a bovine rhodopsin gene as a probe, they found that it bound strongly to one segment of human DNA and less strongly to three other DNA segments. The segment to which the bovine rhodopsin gene bound strongly was shown to be the gene encoding human rhodopsin which resides on chromosome 3 (Sparkes et al 1986, 1987). The three segments to which it bound less strongly were shown to be the genes encoding the colour vision pigments, two (the red and the green colour vision genes) being on the X chromosome and one (the blue colour vision gene) on chromosome 7 (Nathans et al 1986b). Bovine and human rhodopsin are approximately 90% identical in DNA sequence (Nathans & Hogness 1983, 1984), human rhodopsin and colour pigments are approximately 40% identical (Nathans & Hogness 1984), while the red and green pigments show only 43% identity with the blue pigment but 96% mutual identity (Nathans et al 1986a). The fact that the genes encoding the red and green pigments are 96% identical and are located at the end of the long arm of the X chromosome suggests that they arose by a duplication event that occurred recently (in evolutionary terms).

One unexpected finding was that while males with normal colour vision have one red pigment gene on each X chromosome, the number of green pigment genes varied from one to three (Nathans et al 1986a), while occasionally there can even be four or more green pigment genes (Drummond-Borg et al 1987).

Nathans and his colleagues then studied individuals with the four classes of red and green colour blindness. Individuals with deuteranopia were found to have a normal red pigment gene but no green pigment gene(s). Those with protanopia lacked a normal red pigment gene which was replaced by a hybrid red–green pigment gene, and had no green pigment gene or a variable number of them. Deuteranomalous trichromats had a normal red pigment gene, a hybrid red–green gene, with or without normal gene pigment genes. Protanomalous trichromats had no normal red pigment gene, a hybrid red–green pigment gene and a variable number of green pigment genes. These findings were explained by unequal crossovers that resulted in the deletion of a pigment gene or the production of different fusion genes consisting of varying portions of the red and green pigment genes (Nathans et al 1986b, Vollrath et al 1988). Individuals with protanopia and protanomaly appear to have the same genotype (one red–green fusion gene and one intact green gene). Their phenotypic differences could be due to slight differences in the crossover points between the red and green pigment genes, resulting in protein pigments with different in vivo light sensitivity, causing different colour perception (Drummond-Borg et al 1988). Similarly, differences in crossover points could explain the variations that have been described in the degree of impairment in individuals with anomalous trichromacy (protanomaly and deuteranomaly). The molecular methods used up to the present are unable to distinguish between small differences in the position of crossover points.

Blue cone monochromatism

Affected males with this uncommon condition typically present with poor vision from infancy, nystagmus that tends to reduce in amplitude with age, apparently complete or almost complete colour blindness, variable degrees of myopia and astigmatism 'with the rule' (Blackwell & Blackwell 1961, Spivey 1965, Alpern et al 1971, Smith et al 1983).

In three kindreds, tight linkage was found between blue cone monochromatism and two RFLP loci, DXS52 and DXS15, both at Xq28 (Lewis et al 1987), a band on which the red and green colour genes are known to be located (Nathans et al 1986a, 1986b). Abnormalities have been demonstrated in the red and green visual pigment gene cluster, either an unequal homologous recombination and point mutation or a deletion of a 579-bp region upstream of the red pigment gene, which appears to be essential for the activity of both pigment genes (Nathans et al 1989). Further studies of this rare form of monochromatism may throw additional light on the mechanism of colour vision in man.

LEBER'S HEREDITARY OPTIC NEUROPATHY (LHON)

LHON is an uncommon hereditary disorder presenting most commonly in young adult males, but occurring in both sexes and at almost any age, and characterized by the rapid onset of visual failure affecting both eyes within a few weeks of each other. In the acute stage the optic discs are swollen and hyperaemic; in the end stage they are flat and pale. The disorder has been a puzzle and a fascination to ophthalmologists and geneticists for many years. Its hereditary nature has been in no doubt since the original description by Leber in 1871, although the pattern of inheritance, which does not follow Mendelian principles, has until recently been difficult to explain. Our understanding of the disease increased when it became apparent that LHON was transmitted through females mainly to their sons, the sons themselves never passing the disease to their offspring. Another advance occurred when it was shown that most of the offspring of carrier females had a characteristic fundus abnormality, peripapillary microangiopathy (Nikoskelainen et al 1982). This abnormality is present in most daughters and sons of a female carrier, thus satisfying the criteria for a maternally inherited disorder (Nikoskelainen et al 1987).

One possible explanation for maternal inheritance is the occurrence of a mutant gene on the mitochondrial chromosome. Mitochondria contain several copies of a small circular DNA molecule, which in humans consists of 16 569 bp. Mitochondrial DNA differs from DNA in the cell nucleus in being transmitted exclusively by mothers. The most important function of mitochondrial DNA is that it helps to code for a number of enzyme complexes involved in the process of oxidative phosphorylation. It was inevitable, therefore, that a search was made for a mutation in mitochondrial

DNA in patients with LHON, and it was exciting when a mutation was found.

A specific alteration in mitochondrial DNA resulting in a single amino acid substitution has been described as being unique to nine out of 11 families with Leber's optic neuropathy (Wallace et al 1988). This mutation converts a highly conserved arginine residue, at position 11 778, to a histidine in the gene for part of Complex I of the respiratory chain. In another series, this mutation was found in only four out of eight families, and was associated with a poor prognosis for visual recovery; four of five affected males without the 11 778 mutation regained useful vision (Holt et al 1989). All but one of the subjects had a variable mixture of mutant and normal mitochondrial DNA, the relative proportions appearing to be correlated with the risk of developing or transmitting LHON. In another study, the results suggested that different mutations in the genes coding for subunits of Complex I may be the cause of the neuropathy (Vilkki et al 1989), a suggestion supported by the finding of a reduction in mitochondrial electron transport activity in four affected patients (Parker et al 1989). It seems likely that more than one mutation in the mitochondrial DNA may result in LHON.

The substitution of histidine for arginine in a gene coding for a subunit of Complex I is relatively conservative and may result in only a partial reduction in the mitochondrial production of energy. This would result in an energy deficit similar to that caused by potassium cyanide, a known inhibitor of Complex I activity, and it is possible that this energy deficit could be exacerbated by cyanide.

The strong male bias in LHON cannot be explained by a single mitochondrial gene defect alone. The suggestion of an interaction between a mitochondrial gene defect and an X-linked gene coding for an optic nerve isozyme (Wallace 1987) has not, however, been supported by multipoint linkage analysis (Chen et al 1989). The difficulties in diagnosing LHON in females with no apparent family history have recently been emphasized (Franks & Sanders 1990) and may go some way towards explaining the apparent male preponderance in Leber's optic neuropathy. This is, however, just one of the questions still to be answered in this fascinating disorder.

RETINOBLASTOMA

One of the most exciting and fundamentally important advances in ophthalmic genetics has been our increasing understanding of the genetics of cancer as demonstrated by the story of retinoblastoma, the retinoblastoma gene (Rb) now being regarded as the prototype of a class of tumour suppressor genes (anti-oncogenes) whose presence in normal cells is required to prevent the occurrence of a tumour. It has been known for a number of years that retinoblastoma is most commonly a unilateral tumour and, when unilateral, is usually sporadic (without a family history). Less commonly, retinoblastoma is bilateral and then there is often a family history of other affected members, the mode of transmission being autosomal dominant.

That retinoblastoma has a genetic basis was supported by the observation that a small percentage of tumours were associated with a deletion of part of a chromosome belonging to the D group (chromosomes 13–15) (Lele et al 1963). This observation was confirmed by many others and, with improved banding techniques, it became apparent that the deletion involved the long arm of chromosome 13. It is now known that about 4% of Rb patients carry this deletion (Cowell et al 1986). The extent of the deletion varies between cases and, when large, is associated with other congenital anomalies, including mental retardation, cranial and facial abnormalities, anomalies of the fingers and male genital malformations. In each of these cases the deleted band common to all was 13q14 (Yunis & Ramsay 1978). In addition, similar deletions have been found in the cells of some tumours from patients with a normal karyotype.

Additional confirmation of the retinoblastoma predisposition gene being located in band 13q14 came from studies of the enzyme esterase-D (ESD), the locus of which is also on chromosome 13 (van Heyningen et al 1975). Patients with retinoblastoma associated with a deletion, however small, of chromosome 13 usually have an ESD level about 50% of normal and this indicates that the loci for Rb and ESD are closely linked on band 13q14. ESD is a polymorphism with two common variants, ESD1 and ESD2, although ESD1 is much more common than ESD2 in Britain. Because ESD and Rb are so closely linked, the ESD polymorphism can be used to track the inheritance of the Rb gene in informative families and thus make the prenatal diagnosis of retinoblastoma (Fig. 11.7). However, because of the low incidence of the ESD2 allele, only about 10% of families in Britain are at present informative for this polymorphism.

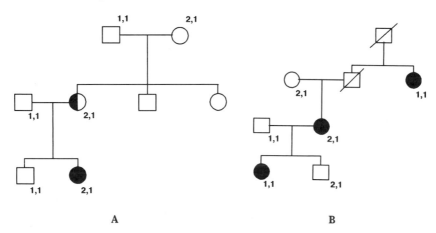

Fig. 11.7 Pedigrees of two families with hereditary retinoblastoma, showing linkage between the retinoblastoma and ESD genes. In family **A** the retinoblastoma gene is closely linked to ESD2, while in family **B** it is linked to ESD1.

Although the predisposition to retinoblastoma is transmitted as an autosomal dominant trait, it is now known that tumour formation results from a recessive mechanism involving the occurrence of two mutant tumour-suppressor genes. The observation that hereditary cases are usually bilateral, multifocal and have an earlier age of onset than unilateral cases, which are usually sporadic and unifocal, led Knudson (1971) to propose that only two mutational events were necessary for tumour formation. In this 'two hit' hypothesis it was postulated that in hereditary retinoblastoma the first mutational event would be inherited through the germ line and be present in every retinal cell, while in sporadic retinoblastoma it would be a somatic mutation in one of the retinal cells. In both types of retinoblastoma the second mutational event would occur somatically and the tumour would develop in any doubly mutant retinal cell. It has now been shown that loss of the second allele in tumour cells often involves loss of a large piece of chromosome 13, resulting either from non-disjunction or from mitotic recombination (Hansen & Cavanee 1988).

After the Rb locus was mapped to band 13q14 it was then necessary to isolate the gene. A chromosome 13 lambda phage library was constructed, the source of the chromosome 13 DNA sequences being either a fluorescence-activated cell sorter (Lalande et al 1984) or rodent/human somatic cell hybrids (Friend et al 1986). Having found one sequence which could detect deletions involving 13q14, chromosome walking techniques were then used to map the surrounding genomic DNA. One of the single copy fragments generated during the chromosome walk recognized a DNA sequence in the mouse genome and in human chromosome 13, suggesting that this fragment contains a coding exon of a gene. This fragment was then used to isolate a cDNA sequence 4.7 kb in length that was present in all normal cells but structurally altered in 30% of retinoblastomas (Friend et al 1986). This work has been confirmed by others (Lee et al 1987, Fung et al 1987) and it is now accepted that 4.7R represents the retinoblastoma predisposition gene. It is a complex gene and consists of 27 exons scattered over a region of about 200 kb (Wiggs et al 1988, Hong et al 1989).

Patients who survive the heritable form of retinoblastoma are at greatly increased risk of developing osteosarcoma and, interestingly, the Rb gene has been found to be deleted in some osteosarcomas. It would appear that homozygous loss of the Rb gene can result in retinoblastoma if the loss of the second allele occurs in the embryonic retina, and in osteosarcoma if the second mutation occurs in bone tissue. Similar changes have been found in a percentage of cell lines from breast cancer (Lee et al 1988) and from small cell lung cancer. The latter tumour does not appear to have a hereditary component and it has been suggested that the Rb gene may be particularly susceptible to carcinogens in tobacco smoke (Harbour et al 1988). Continuing research in this area will help us understand the development of second primary tumours in patients who have had a retinoblastoma, and the occurrence of some primary tumours in relatives of retinoblastoma patients.

CONCLUSIONS

Using several ophthalmic disorders as our examples, we have indicated some of the advances that are occurring in our understanding of the genetic basis of disease. In XLRP, the gene locus was mapped to the short arm of the X chromosome by linkage studies involving restriction fragment length polymorphisms. Shortly afterwards a second locus on the short arm was demonstrated by deletion mapping and further linkage studies. In similar studies, the gene locus for choroideremia was assigned to the proximal long arm of the X chromosome by linkage to RFLPs, and by studying patients with small deletions involving the choroideremia locus. As a result of these advances, more accurate genetic counselling and prenatal diagnosis are now possible in many families with these two disorders.

Using the bovine rhodopsin gene as a probe, the genes encoding human rhodopsin and the colour vision pigments have been isolated and sequenced. These studies have confirmed the hypothesis that rhodopsin and the cone pigments all evolved from a common ancestor and, as a result, contain similar sequences of nucleotides. These advances have increased our understanding of the physiology of colour vision and of its defects.

The pattern of inheritance in Leber's hereditary optic neuropathy can now be explained by mutations in mitochondrial DNA, mitochondria being transmitted exclusively by mothers. The variation in severity and the strong male bias in this disorder have yet to be completely understood.

In retinoblastoma, Knudson's 'two hit' hypothesis has been confirmed by demonstrating deletions of the retinoblastoma gene, or of ESD closely linked to it, in many patients with the tumour, and loss of the second allele in tumour cells indicated by loss of parts of chromosome 13. The retinoblastoma predisposition gene has been isolated by methods including deletion studies and chromosome walking techniques. These advances are of fundamental importance in our understanding of the genetics of cancer and are being applied to a number of other cancers in different organs.

These advances have opened the way to believing that, before long, therapies will become available for many of these genetically determined disorders.

REFERENCES

Alpern M, Lee G B, Maaseidvaag F et al 1971 Colour vision in blue-cone 'monochromacy'. J Physiol 212: 211–233

Barlow D 1989 Pulsed field gel electrophoresis. Genome 31: 465–467

Barrett D J, Bateman J B, Sparkes R S et al 1987 Chromosomal localization of human ornithine aminotransferase gene sequences to 10q26 and Xp11.2. Invest Ophthalmol Vis Sci 28: 1035–1042

Bhattacharya S S, Wright A F, Clayton J F et al 1984 Close genetic linkage between X-linked retinitis pigmentosa and a restriction fragment length polymorphism identified by recombinant DNA probe L1.28. Nature 309: 253–255

Blackwell H R, Blackwell O M 1961 Rod and cone receptor mechanisms in typical and atypical congenital achromatopsia. Vision Res 1: 62–107

Bleeker-Wagemakers L, Friedrich U, Gal A et al 1985 Close linkage between Norrie disease, a cloned DNA sequence from the proximal short arm, and the centromere of the X chromosome. Hum Genet 71: 211–214

Bundey S, Crews S J 1984 A study of retinitis pigmentosa in the city of Birmingham. II. Clinical and genetic heterogeneity. J Med Genet 21: 421–428

Chen J D, Cox I, Denton M J 1989 Preliminary exclusion of an X-linked gene in Leber optic atrophy by linkage analysis. Hum Genet 82: 203–207

Cowell J K, Rutland P, Jay M, Hungerford J 1986 Deletions of the esterase-D locus from a survey of 200 retinoblastoma patients. Hum Genet 72: 164–167

Cremers F P M, Brunsmann F, van de Pol T J R et al 1987 Deletion of the DXS165 locus in patients with classical choroideremia. Clin Genet 32: 421–423

Cremers F P M, van de Pol D J R, Diergaarde P J et al 1989 Physical fine mapping of the choroideremia locus using Xq21 deletions associated with complex syndromes. Genomics 4: 41–46

Cremers F P M, Sankila E-M, Brunsmann F et al 1990 Deletions in patients with classical choroideremia vary in size from 45 kb to several megabases. Am J Hum Genet 47: 622–628

Davies K E (ed) 1988 Genome analysis: a practical approach. IRL Press, Oxford

Davies K E, Young B D, Elles R G et al 1981 Cloning of a representative library of the human X chromosome after sorting by flow cytometry. Nature 293: 374–376

de la Chapelle A, Sankila E M, Lindlof M et al 1985 Norrie disease caused by a gene deletion allowing carrier detection and prenatal diagnosis. Clin Genet 28: 317–320

Denton M J, Chen J D, Serravalle S et al 1988 Analysis of linkage relationships of X-linked retinitis pigmentosa with the following Xp loci: L1.28, OTC, XJ-1.1, pERT87, and C7. Hum Genet 78: 60–64

Drummond-Borg M, Deeb S, Motulsky A G 1987 Molecular detection of color vision anomalies. Am J Hum Genet 41: A96

Drummond-Borg M, Deeb S, Motulsky A G 1988 Molecular basis of abnormal red–green color vision: a family with three types of color vision defects. Am J Hum Genet 43: 675–683

Forrest S M, Smith T J, Kenwrick S J et al 1987 Genetic and physical mapping of markers localised Xp11.0-Xp22.3 on the human X chromosome. Ninth International Workshop on Human Gene Mapping (HGM9) Cytogenet Cell Genet 46: 615

Francke U, Ochs H D, de Martinville B et al 1985 Minor Xp21 chromosome deletion in a male associated with expression of Duchenne muscular dystrophy, chronic granulomatous disease, retinitis pigmentosa, and McLeod syndrome. Am J Hum Genet 37: 250–267

Franks W A, Sanders M D 1990 Leber's hereditary optic neuropathy in women. Eye 4: 482–485

Friedrich U, Warburg M, Wieacker P et al 1985 X-linked retinitis pigmentosa: linkage with the centromere and a cloned DNA sequence from the proximal short arm of the X chromosome. Hum Genet 71: 93–99

Friend S H, Bernards R, Rogelj S et al 1986 A human DNA segment with properties of the gene that predisposes to retinoblastoma and osteosarcoma. Nature 323: 643–646

Fung Y-K T, Murphree A L, T'Ang A et al 1987 Structural evidence for the authenticity of the human retinoblastoma gene. Science 236: 1657–1661

Gal A, Bleeker-Wagemakers L, Wienker T F et al 1985a Localization of the gene for Norrie disease by linkage to the DXS7 locus. Cytogenet Cell Genet 40: 633

Gal A, Stolzenberger C, Wienker T F et al 1985b Norrie's disease: close linkage with genetic markers from the proximal short arm of the X chromosome. Clin Genet 27: 282–283

Gal A, Wieringa B, Smeets D F C M et al 1986 Submicroscopic interstitial deletion of the X chromosome explains a complex syndrome dominated by Norrie disease. Cytogenet Cell Genet 42: 219–224

Gal A, Schinzel A, Orth U et al 1989 Gene of X-chromosomal congenital stationary night blindness is closely linked to DXS7 on Xp. Hum Genet 81: 315–318

Gitschier J, Drayna D, Tuddenhan E G D et al 1985 Genetic mapping and diagnosis of haemophilia A achieved through a BclI polymorphism in the factor VIII gene. Nature 314: 738–740

Hansen M F, Cavanee W K 1988 Retinoblastoma and the progression of tumor genetics. Trends Genet 4: 125–128

Harbour J W, Lai S L, Whang P J et al 1988 Abnormalities in structure and expression of the human retinoblastoma gene in SCLC. Science 241: 353–357

Hodgson S, Robertson M E, Fear C N et al 1987 Prenatal diagnosis of X-linked choroideremia with mental retardation, associated with a cytologically detectable X-chromosome deletion. Hum Genet 75: 286–290

Holt I J, Miller D H, Harding A E 1989 Genetic heterogeneity and mitochondrial DNA heteroplasmy in Leber's hereditary optic neuropathy. J Med Genet 26: 739–743

Hong F D, Huang H-J S, To H et al 1989 Structure of the human retinoblastoma gene. Proc Natl Acad Sci USA 86: 5502–5506

Human Gene Mapping 9 (HGM9) 1987 Cytogenet Cell Genet 46: 1–762

Jay M 1982 On the heredity of retinitis pigmentosa. Br J Ophthalmol 66: 405–416

Jeffreys A J, Wilson V, Thein S L 1985 Hypervariable minisatellite regions in human DNA. Nature 314: 67–73

Katayama S, Wohlferd M, Golbus M S 1988 First demonstration of recombination between the gene for Norrie disease and probe L1.28. Am J Med Genet 30: 967–970

Kingston H M 1989 ABC of clinical genetics. British Medical Association, London

Kivlin J D, Sanborn G E, Wright E et al 1987 Further linkage data on Norrie disease. Am J Med Genet 26: 733–736

Knudson A G Jr 1971 Mutation and cancer: statistical study of retinoblastoma. Proc Natl Acad Sci USA 68: 820–823

Lalande M, Dryja T P, Schreck R R et al 1984 Isolation of human chromosome 13-specific DNA sequences cloned from flow sorted chromosomes and potentially linked to the retinoblastoma locus. Cancer Genet Cytogenet 13: 283–295

Lan N C, Heinzmann C, Gal A et al 1989 Human monoamine oxidase A and B genes map to Xp11.23 and are deleted in a patient with Norrie disease. Genomics 4: 552–559

Leber T 1871 Ueber hereditare und congenital angelegte Sehnervenleiden. Graefes Arch Clin Exp Ophthalmol 2: 249–291

Lee E Y-H P, To H, Shew J-Y et al 1988 Inactivation of the retinoblastoma susceptibility gene in human breast cancers. Science 241: 218–221

Lee W H, Shew J Y, Hong F D et al 1987 The retinoblastoma susceptibility gene encodes a nuclear phosphoprotein associated with DNA binding activity. Nature 329: 642–645

Lele K P, Penrose L S, Stallard H B 1963 Chromosome deletion in a case of retinoblastoma. Ann Hum Genet 27: 171–174

Lesko J G, Lewis R A, Nussbaum R L 1987 Multipoint linkage analysis of loci in the proximal long arm of the human X chromosome: application to mapping the choroideremia locus. Am J Hum Genet 40: 303–311

Lewis R A, Holcomb J D, Bromley W C et al 1987 Mapping X-linked ophthalmic diseases. III. Provisional assignment of the locus for blue cone monochromacy to Xq28. Arch Ophthalmol 105: 1055–1059

MacDonald I M, Sandre R M, Hunter A G W et al 1987 Gene mapping of X-linked choroideremia with restriction fragment-length polymorphisms. Can J Ophthalmol 22: 310–315

Merry D E, Lesko J G, Sosnoski D M et al 1989 Choroideremia and deafness with stapes fixation: a contiguous gene deletion syndrome in Xp21. Am J Hum Genet 45: 530–540

Miyake Y, Yagasaki U, Horiguchi M et al 1986 Congenital stationary night blindness with negative electroretinogram: a new classification. Arch Ophthalmol 104: 1013–1020

Musarella M A, Anson-Cartwright L, Burghes A et al 1989a Linkage analysis of a large

Latin-American family with X-linked retinitis pigmentosa and metallic sheen in the heterozygote carrier. Genomics 4: 601–605

Musarella M A, Weleber R G, Murphey W H et al 1989b Assignment of the gene for complete X-linked congenital stationary night blindness (CSNB1) to Xp11.3. Genomics 5: 727–737

Nathans J, Hogness D S 1983 Isolation, sequence analysis, and intron–exon arrangement of the gene encoding bovine rhodopsin. Cell 34: 807–814

Nathans J, Hogness D S 1984 Isolation and nucleotide sequence of the gene encoding human rhodopsin. Proc Natl Acad Sci USA 81: 4851–4855

Nathans J, Thomas D, Hogness D S 1986a Molecular genetics of human color vision: the genes encoding blue, green, and red pigments. Science 232: 193–202

Nathans J, Piantanida T P, Eddy R L et al 1986b Molecular genetics of inherited variation in human color vision. Science 232: 203–210

Nathans J, Davenport C M, Maumenee I H et al 1989 Molecular genetics of human blue cone monochromacy. Science 25: 831–838

Nikoskelainen E, Hoyt W F, Nummelin K 1982 Ophthalmoscopic findings in Leber's hereditary optic neuropathy: I. Fundus findings in asymptomatic family members. Arch Ophthalmol 100: 1597–1602

Nikoskelainen E K, Savontaus M-L, Wanne O P et al 1987 Leber's hereditary optic neuroretinopathy, a maternally inherited disease: a genealogic study in four pedigrees. Arch Ophthalmol 105: 665–671

Ngo J T, Spence M A, Cortessis V et al 1988a Recombinational event between Norrie disease and DXS7 loci. Clin Genet 34: 43–47

Ngo J T, Bateman J B, Cortessis V et al 1988b Norrie disease: linkage analysis using the L1.28 and the human ornithine-aminotransferase (OAT) cDNA probes. In: Piatigorsky J, Shinohara T, Zelenka P S (eds) Molecular biology of the eye: genes, vision, and ocular disease. Liss, New York, pp 329–338

Ngo J T, Bateman J B, Cortessis V et al 1989 Norrie disease: linkage analysis using a 4.2-kb RFLP detected by a human ornithine aminotransferase cDNA probe. Genomics 4: 539–545

Nussbaum R L, Lewis R A, Lesko J G et al 1985a Mapping ophthalmological disease. II. Linkage of relationship of X-linked retinitis pigmentosa to X chromosome short arm markers. Hum Genet 70: 45–50

Nussbaum R L, Lewis R A, Lesko J G et al 1985b Choroideremia is linked to the restriction fragment length polymorphism DXYS1 at Xq13–21. Am J Hum Genet 37: 473–481

Nussbaum R L, Lesko J G, Lewis R A et al 1987 Isolation of anonymous DNA sequences from within a submicroscopic X chromosomal deletion in a patient with choroideremia, deafness, and mental retardation. Proc Natl Acad Sci USA 84: 6521–6525

Ott J 1986 A short guide to linkage analysis. In: Davies K E (ed) Human genetic diseases: a practical approach. IRL Press, Oxford, pp 19–32

Parker W D Jr, Oley C A, Parks J K 1989 A defect in mitochondrial electron-transport activity (NADH-coenzyme Q oxidoreductase) in Leber's hereditary optic neuropathy. N Engl J Med 320: 1331–1333

Redmond R M, Graham C A, Craig I W et al 1990 DNA analysis and recombination in X-linked retinitis pigmentosa. Eye 4: 204–209

Roberts R J 1985 Restriction enzymes. In: Hames B D, Higgins S J (eds) Nucleic acid hybridisation: a practical approach. IRL Press, Oxford, pp 203–210

Ruddle F H 1981 A new era in mammalian gene mapping: somatic cell genetics and recombinant DNA methodologies. Nature 294: 115–120

Saiki R K, Gelfand D H, Stoffel S et al 1988 Primer-directed enzymatic amplification of DNA with a thermostable DNA polymerase. Science 239: 487–491

Saint-Basile G de, Bohler M C, Fischer A et al 1988 Xp21 DNA microdeletion in a patient with chronic granulomatous disease, retinitis pigmentosa, and Mcleod phenotype. Hum Genet 80: 85–89

Sankila E-M, de La Chapelle A, Karna J et al 1987 Choroideremia: close linkage to DXYS1 and DXYS12 demonstrated by segregation analysis and historical–genealogical evidence. Clin Genet 31: 315–322

Schwartz M, Rosenberg T, Niebuhr E et al 1986 Choroideremia: further evidence for assignment of the locus to Xq13–Xq21. Hum Genet 74: 449–452

Smith V C, Pokorny J, Delleman J W et al 1983 X-linked incomplete achromatopsia with more than one class of functional cones. Invest Ophthalmol Vis Sci 24: 451–457

Southern E M 1975 Detection of specific sequences among DNA fragments separated by gel electrophoresis. J Mol Biol 98: 503–517

Sparkes R S, Mohandas T, Newman S L et al 1986 Assignment of the rhodopsin gene to human chromosome 3. Invest Ophthalmol Vis Sci 27: 1170–1172

Sparkes R S, Klisak I, Kaufman D et al 1987 Assignment of the rhodopsin gene to human chromosome three, region 3q21–3q24 by in-situ hybridization studies. Curr Eye Res 5: 797–798

Spivey B E 1965 The X-linked recessive inheritance of atypical monochromatism. Arch Ophthalmol 74: 327–333

van Heyningen V, Bobrow M, Bodmer W F et al 1975 Chromosome assignment of some human enzyme loci: mitochondrial malate dehydrogenase to 7, mannosphosphate isomerase and pyruvate kinase to 15, and probably, esterase-d to 13. Ann Hum Genet 38: 295–303

Vilkki J, Savontaus M-L, Kalimo H et al 1989 Mitochondrial DNA polymorphism in Finnish families with Leber's hereditary optic neuroretinopathy. Hum Genet 82: 208–212

Vollrath D, Nathans J, Davis R W 1988 Tandem array of human visual pigment genes at Xq28. Science 240: 1669–1672

Wallace D C 1987 Maternal genes: mitochondrial diseases. Birth Defects 23: 137–190

Wallace D C, Singh G, Lott M T et al 1988 Mitochondrial DNA mutation associated with Leber's hereditary optic neuropathy. Science 242: 1427–1430

Wallace R B, Schold M, Johnson M J et al 1981 Oligonucleotide directed mutagenesis of the human beta-globin gene: a general method for producing specific point mutations in cloned DNA. Nucleic Acids Res 9: 3647–3656

Weatherall D J 1985 The new genetics and clinical practice, 2nd edn. Oxford University Press, Oxford

Wiggs J, Nordenskjold M, Yandell D et al 1988 Prediction of the risk of hereditary retinoblastoma using DNA polymorphisms within the retinoblastoma gene. N Engl J Med 318: 151–157

Yunis J J, Ramsay N 1978 Retinoblastoma and subband deletion of chromosome 13. Am J Dis Child 132: 161–163

Index